VASCULAR SURGERY

MODERN NURSING SERIES

General Editors
A. J. HARDING RAINS M.S., F.R.C.S.
Professor of Surgery, Charing Cross Hospital Medical School
Honorary Consultant Surgeon, Charing Cross Hospital

MISS VALERIE HUNT S.R.N., S.C.M., R.N.T.
District Nursing Officer, Avon Health Authority (Teaching)

This Series caters for the needs of a wide range of nursing, medical and ancillary professions. Some of the titles are given below, but a complete list is available from the Publisher.

Neurology
EDWIN R. BICKERSTAFF M.D., F.R.C.P.

Venereology and Genito-Urinary Medicine
R. D. CATTERALL F.R.C.P.(EDIN.)

Obstetrics and Gynaecology
JOAN M. E. QUIXLEY S.R.N., R.N.T.
MICHAEL D. CAMERON M.A., M.B., B.CHIR., F.R.C.S., F.R.O.G.

Rheumatology
D. R. SWINSON M.B., B.S., M.R.C.P.
W. R. SWINBURN M.B., M.R.C.P.

Principles of Medicine and Medical Nursing
J. C. HOUSTON M.D., F.R.C.P.
HILARY HYDE WHITE S.R.N.

Microbiology in Patient Care
H. I. WINNER M.D., M.R.C.P., F.R.C.PATH.

**The Older Patient
a textbook of geriatrics**
R. E. IRVINE M.A., M.D., F.R.C.P.
M. K. BAGNALL A.I.S.W.
B. J. SMITH S.R.N., R.F.N.

Principles of Surgery and Surgical Nursing
SELWYN TAYLOR D.M., M.CH., F.R.C.S.

Emergency and Acute Care
A. J. HARDING RAINS M.S., F.R.C.S.
VALERIE HUNT S.R.N., R.N.T.
KEITH REYNOLDS M.S., F.R.C.S.

Therapeutics
J. G. LEWIS M.D., F.R.C.P.

Ear, Nose and Throat Surgery and Nursing
R. PRACY M.B., B.S., F.R.C.S.
J. SIEGLER M.B., B.S., D.L.O., F.R.C.S.
P. M. STELL M.B., F.R.C.S.
J. ROGERS M.A., F.R.C.A.

Textbook of Medicine
R. J. HARRISON CH.B., M.D.

VASCULAR SURGERY

R. E. HORTON
M.B.E., M.S., F.R.C.S.(ENG.)
Consultant Surgeon, United Bristol Hospitals

HODDER AND STOUGHTON
LONDON SYDNEY AUCKLAND TORONTO

LQM JGJ

British Library Cataloguing in Publication Data

Horton, R. E.
  Vascular surgery. – (Modern nursing series).
  1. Blood-vessels – Surgery
  I. Title II. Series
  617′.413   RD598

ISBN 0 340 22495 9 Boards
ISBN 0 340 22496 7 Unibook Pbk

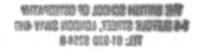
First published 1980

Printed and bound in Great Britain
for Hodder and Stoughton Educational
a division of Hodder and Stoughton Ltd.,
Mill Road, Dunton Green, Sevenoaks, Kent,
by Richard Clay (The Chaucer Press), Ltd.,
Bungay, Suffolk.

Editors' Foreword

The scope of this series has increased since it was first established, and it now serves a wide range of medical, nursing and ancillary professions, in line with the present trend towards the belief that all who care for patients in a clinical context have an increasing amount in common.

The texts are carefully prepared and organized so that they may be readily kept up to date as the rapid developments of medical science demand. The series already includes many popular books on various aspects of medical and nursing care, and reflects the increased emphasis on community care.

The increasing specialization in the medical profession is fully appreciated and the books are often written by Physicians or Surgeons in conjunction with specialist nurses. For this reason, they will not only cover the syllabus of training of the General Nursing Council, but will be designed to meet the needs of those undertaking training controlled by the Joint Board of Clinical Studies set up in 1970.

Preface

In the twenty-five years that I have been concerned with vascular surgery it has developed from a somewhat experimental and dangerous branch of surgery to a recognized specialty which is routinely practised in District Hospitals throughout the world with safety and great benefit to the patients.

Vascular surgery is sometimes presented in textbooks of cardio-vascular surgery where it tends to take second place to cardiac surgery. In this work I have attempted to describe and illustrate vascular surgery in simple terms. The illustrations are confined to line drawings which are easy to interpret. The book is primarily intended for nurses but it may also be useful for medical students and for those reading for examinations in surgery.

I wish to acknowledge my thanks to Margaret Sutton for her advice and help, and to Judy Coppin who typed and re-typed the script and assisted me with the text.

The original diagram illustrating the sympathetic nervous system was drawn by Mr. E. J. Turnbull.

Bristol, 1980   R. E. H.

Contents

Part 1

Surgery of the Peripheral Arteries

1
Acute Ischaemia

Ischaemia means reduction of blood supply to a part of the body, and when this is sudden, dramatic and complete it is referred to as acute ischaemia. Acute ischaemia of a limb is one of the great surgical emergencies.

Causes of Acute Ischaemia

Acute ischaemia is due to the sudden occlusion of a major artery so suddenly preventing the flow of blood to that part.

Embolism. In this condition the acute ischaemia is caused by a clot of blood (a thrombus) which has previously been formed in a cavity of the heart or on a patch of atheroma in an artery—see below—and which suddenly becomes detached and is swept along in the blood stream. It is arrested when it reaches a vessel too small for it to pass any further, and the circulation is arrested at this point.

Trauma. An accident may involve a major artery and so cause acute ischaemia beyond the point of injury.

Atherosclerosis. In atherosclerosis there is a gradual narrowing of the artery because of the deposition of plaques of yellow tissue (called atheroma) in the wall of the artery. As the process of narrowing is a gradual one other blood vessels called collaterals (Fig. 1.1) usually develop, so that when the main artery finally closes there are no signs of acute ischaemia. However, sometimes the collateral circulation does not develop adequately and acute ischaemia develops when thrombosis occurs in the artery.

Signs of Acute Ischaemia

It is particularly important for doctors and nurses to be able to recognize acute ischaemia as the treatment is urgent. Sometimes a community or home nurse caring for an elderly person with a bad heart may be the first person to whom the patient complains.

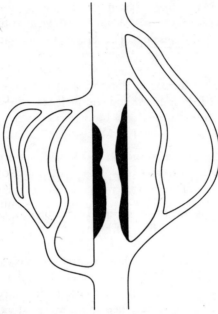

Fig. 1.1 Development of collateral circulation. The main artery is shown narrowed by atherosclerosis. New blood vessels formed to bypass the stenosis are called collaterals.

The first effects of acute ischaemia are upon the peripheral nerves. The part affected becomes anaesthetic as a result of failure of function of the sensory nerves. The nerves are unable to pass impulses from the skin to the brain where sensations are interpreted. Also, because of the interference with function of the motor nerves, the muscles cease to function and the patient is unable to move the ischaemic part. These effects are present within 15 minutes of the arrest of the circulation. When the circulation is restored function returns to the peripheral nerves.

The sudden arrest of inflow of blood causes the part to be emptied of blood so that it appears pale in colour. The skin temperature of a limb is dependent on the flow of blood through the skin. When the flow ceases the temperature begins to fall, but this is a slow process and is to some extent dependent on the temperature of the environment. In a very hot climate cooling may not be noticeable. Later, when there is no inflow of blood and little outflow, the remaining blood stagnating in the skin and losing its oxygen to the tissues becomes blue. So the limb, which is initially pale and warm, gradually becomes blue and cold.

Muscle can remain alive without blood flow for 6–8 hours and after this it undergoes necrosis (death). It is essential to restore the circulation before the muscles die as after this amputation is inevitable.

Treatment of the Acutely Ischaemic Limb

Surgical Treatment

In most cases an operation is urgently indicated to restore the circulation, and the type of operation depends on the cause of the arterial obstruction. For example, an arterial embolus is treated by the operation of removal of the embolus (embolectomy); an injured artery is repaired or replaced with a graft; and an atherosclerotic occlusion is treated with a bypass vein graft.

Medical Treatment

Although the only effective treatment of acute ischaemia is a surgical operation the surgeon may consider such an operation too risky. He may also wish to delay it for some hours to improve the patient's general condition or to see if some recovery of the circulation takes place. During this period certain non-surgical measures are taken.

1. Exposure

There is no strong evidence that this measure is of value but it is customary to expose an ischaemic limb to room temperature while keeping the rest of the body covered. The idea is that the cooled limb will need less oxygen for its survival. The use of fans and other techniques for cooling is now obsolete.

2. Posture

There is no doubt that the blood to an ischaemic limb is affected by posture. It should never be raised as this will still further reduce blood flow. The limb should be lowered below heart level when gravity will assist the flow of blood into the limb. Sometimes it is convenient to put blocks under the head of the bed, but if the patient is in shock this cannot be done and the individual limb must be lowered along the side of the bed where it can be supported on a chair.

3. Anticoagulants

When an artery is occluded the blood below the point of occlusion ceases to flow and this stagnant column of blood tends to thrombose after 5 or 6 hours. If the patient is to be treated conservatively it is wise to use anticoagulants to prevent this thrombosis which is called a propagated thrombus (Fig. 1.2). Intravenous heparin is the most convenient drug and is most commonly used. An intravenous infusion is set up, and after giving 10 000 units i.v. as a loading dose the heparin drip is given at the rate of 20 000 units in 12 hours. A convenient carrier is dextrose and saline.

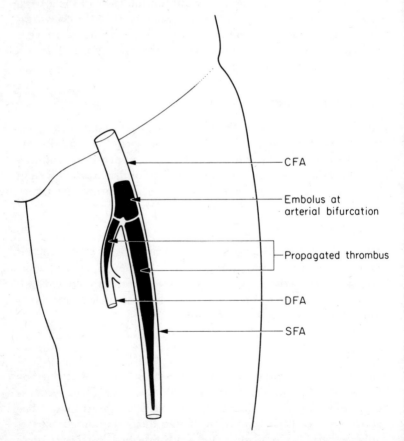

Fig. 1.2 Femoral embolus. The embolus is shown at the femoral bifurcation. Propagated thrombus has formed in the superficial and deep femoral arteries. CFA, common femoral artery; SFA, superficial femoral artery; DFA, deep femoral artery.

4. Low Molecular Weight Dextran

When this substance was first introduced it was thought that the circulatory improvement which resulted was due to reduction of viscosity of the blood enabling it to pass more easily through the capillaries. It is now thought that the effect is simply due to dilution of the blood which is similar to that resulting from the use of intravenous saline but much longer acting.

The usual dose is 500 ml of Dextran in saline given every 12 hours. It is convenient to add 20 000 units of heparin to each bottle of Dextran.

2
Chronic Ischaemia

In this condition there is a reduction of the flow of blood to a part of the body—most commonly a leg—insufficient to give rise to an acute emergency but enough to cause marked symptoms and signs and interference with normal function. The condition of chronic ischaemia may remain stationary for a long time, but over a period of months the blood flow may improve as a result of development of collateral arteries or deteriorate as a result of the gradual advance of the disease process.

Cause of Chronic Ischaemia

Chronic ischaemia is nearly always caused by atherosclerosis which causes gradual narrowing of the arteries. It is a progressive disease, and without treatment the condition is inclined to deteriorate gradually.

Effects of Chronic Ischaemia

1. Intermittent Claudication

The word claudication is derived from a Greek word meaning 'to limp'. Some surgeons prefer to speak of this condition as intermittent limping. The condition arises when there is an obstruction to the main blood supply to the leg. There are no symptoms at rest. When the patient walks and uses his muscles there is a need to increase the flow of blood to the leg. When the main artery is obstructed and the increased flow cannot take place the muscles are unable to function properly. The patient begins to limp because of pain and lack of proper function in his leg muscle, and finally has to stop. The need for an increased blood flow is now over and the pain soon passes enabling the patient to start walking again. The site of pain of intermittent claudication varies according to the site of the arterial obstruction. The calf of the leg is most commonly affected but buttock, thigh, and foot claudication also occur.

Sometimes an occlusion in the main artery to the arm causes similar effects in the forearm which is sufficient to stop a man from using the arm for work.

2. Rest Pain

When the degree of ischaemia is more severe the patient may complain of severe pain in the foot at rest. This may be due to lack of sufficient blood supply to the nerve endings. Rest pain is severe and relentless and impossible to relieve even with the most powerful drugs. Patients with rest pain get no sleep, deteriorate quickly, and ask for an amputation to relieve them. They sometimes discover that the pain is better if the leg is suspended over the bedside at night.

3. Gangrene

In the most severe form of chronic ischaemia the blood supply is so reduced that it is insufficient to maintain life, and there is local tissue death which is called gangrene. This usually begins at the most peripheral part of a toe but may also occur where pressure contributes to the ischaemia at the back of the heel. Death of tissue is called necrosis. When necrosis occurs in some external part of the body it becomes infected with putrefying organisms and this is called gangrene. Most gangrene seen today is dry gangrene in which the part is black, shrivelled, dry and with a faint odour of putrefaction. Wet gangrene is rarely seen except in cases of diabetes. In these cases the infection is a much more prominent and dangerous feature. The part is freely suppurating and the smell is very offensive. Severe rest pain accompanies gangrene.

Treatment of Chronic Ischaemia

Medical Treatment

Patients with arterial disease are often very worried about their condition. Elderly men fear the onset of gangrene and loss of a leg. Doctors and nurses have a duty to try and overcome these fears and to explain the possibilities of modern treatment.

1. Anaemia. If the patient's ability to carry oxygen in the blood is reduced by anaemia this should be corrected. Restoration of the haemoglobin level to normal may lengthen the distance a patient can walk before getting intermittent claudication.

2. Exercise. The patient suffering from intermittent claudication should be encouraged to walk as far as his disability allows. Walking may cause some development of the collateral circulation and eventually increase the walking distance. It is possible for a patient to modify his way of life so that he can live with his disability. For example, he may find that walking at a slower pace he does not have to stop, and re-routing his walk to avoid a slope may also prevent claudication.

3. Smoking. All forms of vascular disease are made worse by smoking, and smoking must be absolutely forbidden.

4. Posture. In patients just beginning to get rest pain some benefit may come from lowering the limb in bed at night. One easy way to do this is to put blocks under the head of the bed so that gravity helps the circulation into the leg.

5. Vasodilator Drugs. Most patients with chronic ischaemia are given vasodilator drugs. There are a great number of these drugs available and all are effective in dilating normal arteries. When given by mouth vasodilator drugs have a generalized effect, but in patients with rigid atherosclerotic arteries the effect in no way matches the vasodilator effect in a normal subject. Experiments show that although the blood flow to a normal limb is increased when vasodilators are used they do not have a comparable effect in cases when the artery is occluded. There is in fact considerable doubt about the wisdom of giving vasodilator drugs in any circumstances.

Surgical Treatment

A variety of operations are used in chronic ischaemia.

Sympathectomy

This operation which removes the sympathetic nerve supply to a part causes a selective vasodilatation of the part of the body selected for the operation. In this way it differs from vasodilator drugs which have a generalized effect.

The sympathetic nervous system does not have any control over muscle circulation so that sympathectomy is valueless in the treatment of intermittent claudication. It may be used to improve the skin circulation but the effect is never dramatic because the rigid vessels found in atherosclerosis do not dilate in the same way as normal arteries.

Sympathetic block may be used in place of the operation of sympathectomy. In this procedure phenol is injected into the sympathetic chain to destroy it.

Artery Grafting

This operation is undoubtedly the most effective way of treating chronic ischaemia. Many cases are suitable for surgical treatment by grafting. When the obstruction is in the aorta or iliac arteries it is usual to use synthetic grafts, and dacron is the most popular material in use for this operation.

Dacron grafts show some tendency to thrombose when used to bypass the smaller arteries in the leg, and for this purpose the long saphenous vein is commonly used. The long saphenous vein has a thick muscular wall and withstands arterial pressure without difficulty. As the vein is fitted with valves to ensure a flow from the foot towards the heart, the piece of vein needed for graft has to be removed and reversed so that the valves do not obstruct the flow of blood.

Endarterectomy

This operation is sometimes popularly referred to as the 'reboring' operation. It depends on the fact that in cases of atheromatous occlusion a plane of cleavage develops in the media which is the middle and main part of the wall of the artery. It is possible for the surgeon to find this plane of cleavage and to extract the atheromatous plaques from the interior of the artery. Special instruments have been devised for this operation and long lengths of atheroma can be removed. When endarterectomy is completed the wall of the artery consists of the adventitia and less than half the media. This is quite strong enough to withstand arterial pressure, but the absence of the lining of intima often results in early thrombosis of the endarterectomized segment especially when the operation is performed on the medium-sized arteries such as the femoral or popliteal. Endarterectomy is more successful when performed on the aorta and iliac arteries.

3

Investigation of Vascular Cases

Arteriography

The most important investigation in cases of arterial disease is radiography. Plain X-ray films may show calcification particularly in cases of atherosclerosis. The surgeon will be interested to know about this as it may cause difficulty with suturing in a graft operation, but calcification is not a contra-indication. In the radiographic investigation called arteriography radio-opaque fluid, usually referred to as dye, is injected into the artery. As the dye is carried distally in the flowing blood stream a series of pictures can be taken which will show the outline of the artery at the point of injection and beyond it. Automatic machines are available to expose X-ray films in rapid succession but if one is not available it can be done manually.

Although arteriography is now a routine and safe investigation patients often show great anxiety. The procedure must be fully explained and the patient assured of the safety and diagnostic value.

The most commonly used techniques concern investigation of the circulation in the legs. This can be done by introducing the dye into the aorta (lumbar aortography) or into the common femoral artery (femoral arteriography).

The carotid arteries and cerebral circulation are frequently investigated by carotid arteriography, and many of the viscera in the abdomen can be investigated and their arteries injected by special techniques. Even the coronary arteries of the heart can be X-rayed and atherosclerotic narrowing or occlusion demonstrated.

As there is a very rapid flow of blood in a large artery it is necessary to inject a large amount of dye very quickly. Small amounts of dye are quickly diluted and lost in the blood stream.

All forms of arteriography carry a slight risk and the investigation should only be done if the surgeon believes that some form of surgical treatment may be done after examination of the radiographs. Toxic reactions to the radio-opaque dye are now very rare. The main difficulties are mechanical. The needle must be placed well inside the artery. If the injection is made when the needle is outside the artery the dye will infiltrate locally and cause pain for some hours. If the bevel of the needle is partly in the aorta and partly in its wall some of the dye may go into the wall of the aorta and damage it. This is the most serious accident that can happen.

When the needle is removed bleeding may take place. To control this pressure is applied to the puncture site with a small sponge and this is kept in place for 5 minutes. This gives sufficient time for platelets from the blood stream to plug the hole made by the needle. Of course this cannot be done with translumbar aortography and some bleeding always takes place and causes some bruising around the aorta. Serious bleeding is very rare but the patient may complain of back pain. After aortography the patient should always be watched carefully for signs of internal haemorrhage. If elevation of the pulse and lowering of the blood pressure occurs with sweating the doctor should be informed immediately.

Lumbar Aortography

This may be done by either of two techniques. A catheter may be introduced through the femoral artery by the Seldinger technique which is described later. The alternative and older technique is to introduce a needle into the aorta from the back.

The patient is anaesthetized and placed in the prone position on the X-ray table. The aortography needle is inserted into the back on the left side and directed towards the body of the third lumbar vertebra (Fig. 3.1 a and b). If the needle strikes the vertebral body it is withdrawn a few centimetres and redirected to pass in front of the body of the vertebra where it will enter the aorta. This is confirmed by the spurting of blood from the needle. The needle is connected to a length of tubing attached to a syringe. The join must be of a locking variety as the high-pressure injection will cause the syringe to separate from the tubing if not securely locked.

When all is ready a trial injection of 6 ml is given and a radiograph taken. If this film shows the needle to be correctly sited within the aorta the full injection of 30 ml of 70% solution is given and a series of X-rays taken down the leg in time with the flow of blood and radio-opaque dye. Generally this is done on an X-ray table which automatically moves the patient headwards for each X-ray.

Arterial Catheterization

In this technique a fine plastic cannula is introduced into the femoral artery at the groin and passed proximally into the aorta. Originally described by Seldinger of Stockholm, this is now generally referred to as the Seldinger technique, although the original technique has been considerably modified and improved.

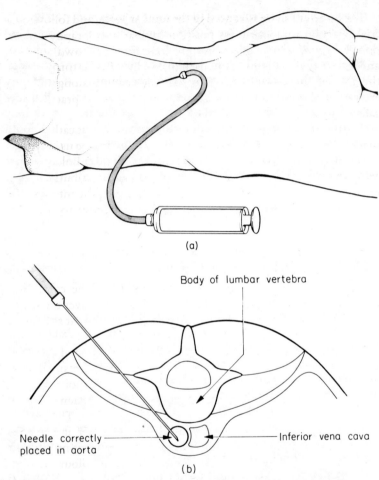

(a)

Body of lumbar vertebra

Needle correctly placed in aorta

Inferior vena cava

(b)

Fig. 3.1 Translumbar aortography. In (a) the position of the needle puncture in the back is shown. In (b) the route is shown to pass the side of the body of the vertebra to enter the aorta which lies in front of the vertebra.

The investigation is usually performed under local anaesthetic on the X-ray table. An image intensifier is used and this is connected to a television screen so that when this is switched on the operator can see the position of the catheter and of any dye which is injected.

A needle is introduced into the femoral artery and a teflon coated guide wire is passed through the needle and proximally towards the aorta. The needle can then be withdrawn over the guide wire which is left in position. The teflon catheter is then threaded over the guide wire until the guide wire appears beyond the catheter. The wire is then pulled out leaving the catheter in the artery.

The catheter can be advanced to the lumbar aorta, and following a trial injection to confirm its position lumbar aortography can be done by giving a large injection and taking films to show the pelvic and leg arteries. In cases of atherosclerosis when there is tortuosity of the arteries it may be difficult to pass the catheter along the iliac arteries, and translumbar aortography may be more practical and safer.

The main advantage of the Seldinger technique is that catheters are made with a variety of shapes at the tip and these can be used to pass the catheter into the main branches of the aorta. The radiologist may catheterize the renal arteries to show the shape and distribution of the renal arteries, the mesenteric artery which supplies the intestine, or the coeliac axis which gives rise to the main arteries to the liver (hepatic artery) and spleen (splenic artery).

Complications of Arterial Catheterization

1. This technique is not without risk. When the catheter is withdrawn firm pressure must be maintained over the site to prevent bleeding. A small aneurysm may form at the site of catheterization.
2. Thrombosis of the artery has followed prolonged catheterization especially in children whose arteries are small. The after-care should therefore include observations on the colour of the limb and other signs of acute ischaemia which might follow thrombosis of the femoral artery. The acutely ischaemic limb is often painful at first. Later it becomes numb and the muscles become paralysed so that movement is impossible. There are usually dramatic colour changes from the pallor to blotchy blueness.
3. In passing the Seldinger catheter through a tortuous and atheromatous artery it is possible to dislodge a plaque of atheroma and this may occlude the artery causing an acutely ischaemic leg and an acute surgical emergency.

Brachial Artery Catheterization

Other arteries such as the brachial artery in the arm may be catheterized. The artery is smaller and the technique more difficult. Complications such as thrombosis are also more likely because of the small size of the artery.

Femoral Arteriography

This is usually performed when the surgeon requires information concerning an occlusion in one leg. It is best performed under general anaesthetic but can be done with a local anaesthetic and sedation. However, the injection under local anaesthetic can be very painful.

The needle is placed in the femoral artery with the patient lying on his back on the X-ray table. The details are similar to those described under lumbar aortography. Following a successful test dose an injection of 20 ml of dye is made and a series of films exposed under the leg (Fig. 3.2).

Carotid Arteriography

In this investigation radio-opaque dye is injected into the common carotid artery in the neck. Sometimes the investigation is done on both sides. This form of arteriography is more dangerous than any other and should only be performed by those familiar with the

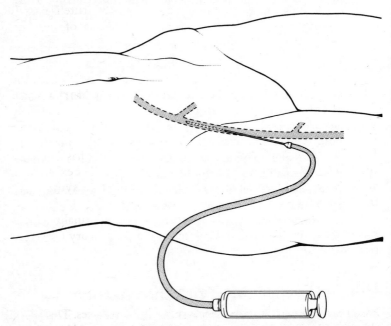

Fig. 3.2 Percutaneous femoral arteriography. The needle is placed in the lumen of the common femoral or external iliac artery after puncturing the artery just below the groin crease.

technique. The serious occasional complication is a stroke (hemiplegia). This may result from too large an injection or the use of a too concentrated form of dye. There is also the risk of dislodging a fragment of thrombus or of injecting a small amount of air. Air consists of various gases but about 79% is nitrogen which is insoluble. If this reaches an important artery in the brain the artery will remain occluded for many hours while the nitrogen is slowly absorbed, and during this time the brain will undergo irreversible damage.

Observations following Arteriography

1. General observations include the pulse rate and blood pressure which should initially be taken every 15 minutes. In addition the patient must be observed for sweating.
2. Local observations at the site of the needle puncture. The nurse should take note of any swelling which is due to haematoma or actual bleeding from the needle puncture.
3. The limb should be observed for signs of acute ischaemia. These include observations on the colour of the limb, abnormal sensations, pain and paralysis.

Other Investigations done on Vascular Cases

Blood Tests

It is usual to estimate the haemoglobin. If the patient has any degree of anaemia the symptoms of a vascular occlusion will be exacerbated, and correction of anaemia may cause considerable symptomatic improvement.

In some cases of atherosclerosis there is an abnormality of lipid metabolism, and blood should be sent to the laboratory for estimation of blood lipids.

Diabetes

Many patients with atherosclerosis suffer from diabetes. This should always be investigated by testing the urine for sugar and ketones and by estimating the fasting blood sugar. In the event of any abnormality it is necessary to do a full glucose tolerance test.

Cardiovascular Tests

As atherosclerosis is a generalized disease it is necessary to direct investigations to other parts of the body which may be affected. The coronary arteries of the heart are frequently affected and narrowing causes cardiac muscle ischaemia and sometimes infarction. This can be detected by electrocardiography (ECG).

Atherosclerosis may be seen in the retinal arteries with the ophthalmoscope.

Pulse Volume Recording

A sphygmomanometer cuff is placed round the leg just above the ankle and is inflated with air. The pulse in the leg causes pressure changes in the air inside the cuff and in the connecting tube. At the end of the tube there is a transducer which converts pressure changes to electrical currents; these are electronically converted to wave forms which are traced on a piece of moving paper. In a normal leg the wave form consists of a sharp vertical upstroke followed by a more gradual fall, but when the circulation is impaired the wave form is much lower and shows a smooth contour. This investigation is used at operation immediately the clamps are removed to confirm that circulation has been restored. It is also done in the recovery room when clinical signs of patency of the graft may be difficult to interpret. The apparatus is easy to use and is well within the capability of nurses.

Doppler Studies (see also p. 138)

The Doppler effect is the change in frequency of a sound wave which occurs when it is reflected from a moving object such as a red blood cell inside an artery. Ultrasound (sound waves which are not audible by the human ear) is used to detect it. The Doppler probe is held over the site of an artery, such as the posterior tibial behind the medial malleolus at the ankle, and the reflected waves are converted in the instrument to audible sound which can then be heard by using earphones. By using an ordinary blood pressure apparatus it is possible to measure the blood pressure in the arteries of the foot. The sound disappears when the cuff is inflated to systolic blood pressure. There are now Doppler scanners which use 30 different sources of ultrasound and using special techniques it is possible to show the size and shape of an artery. The technique is not yet as good as arteriography but it is likely to replace arteriography eventually and has the advantage that it is non-invasive and without any risk.

4
Materials used in Vascular Surgery

Grafts

There are a number of circumstances in vascular surgery in which an occluded segment of blood vessel has to be replaced with a graft. Grafts may be of several kinds both biological and synthetic.

Biological Grafts

Three types of grafts are recognized:

1. Heterograft. A heterograft is a graft taken from an animal of a different species. Unfortunately the protein content of a graft taken from an animal is rejected by the patient and heterografts have not been successful.

2. Homograft. This is a graft taken from an animal of the same species. In the early days of vascular surgery between 1950 and 1960 homografts were extensively used. The arteries were taken from the bodies of young men who had died in accidents, and were stored either at low temperature or at normal temperature after freeze drying. Homografts were difficult to obtain and there were legal and ethical difficulties concerning the removal of grafts from the recently dead. In addition they are subject to rejection and the elastic was gradually replaced by fibrous tissue causing weakness and aneurysm formation in some cases. As a result of these difficulties homografts are now rarely used.

3. Autograft. An autograft is a graft of material taken from the same patient. Of course there is not much scope for using arteries for this technique but a vein, especially the long saphenous vein, may be used as an autograft and used to bypass an occlusion in an artery of the same patient. This is because the saphenous vein is a very muscular tube and well able to withstand arterial pressure. Another reason for the successful outcome of venous grafts is the fact that the autograft is a living graft which is not rejected as it is transferred to a different part of the same patient. Although rejection does not take place the muscle of the graft is gradually replaced by fibrous tissue. Aneurysmal dilation does not take place and autogenous vein grafts have been very successful and often remain patent for many years.

4. Vein Patches. When an artery has to be opened for any purpose its subsequent closure is certain to result in some narrowing. In most cases it is wiser to close the opening in the artery with a patch of vein so that the lumen is not narrowed. Such a patch may be taken from any convenient vein in the arm or leg. Patches made from a sheet of knitted dacron are also used by some surgeons (Fig. 4.1).

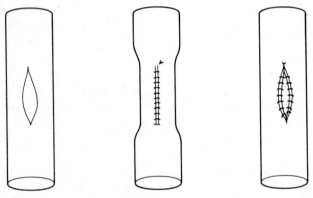

Fig. 4.1 This illustrates the value of a vein patch to prevent narrowing after incision and suture of an artery.

Synthetic Grafts

A good many different types of man-made fibre have been used in the past but at present most synthetic grafts are made of dacron. Grafts are made in tubes of a variety of diameters. A 10 millimetre graft is usually used for iliac and femoral artery grafts. There are also a variety of sizes of bifurcated grafts which are used when the aorta and both iliac arteries have to be replaced. Some grafts have a longitudinal black line to prevent them twisting on insertion.

Graft Weave

Dacron grafts are made with a crimped design. The graft lengthens when arterial pressurized blood is inside and the crimping allows the graft to be curved in the body without kinking.

Two different weaves of dacron are used in the manufacture of grafts. The woven graft is the most commonly used. The knitted graft is less popular as it may bleed more but the suturing properties are better and the cut edge is less likely to fray.

Preclotting of Dacron Grafts

All fibre grafts are porous and need to be preclotted. When the graft is selected about 10 ml of blood is taken from the patient and put into a small dish with the graft. The outside of the graft is thoroughly soaked in blood which clots in the interstices between the weave so preventing leakage of blood when the graft is put into the circulation.

If the surgeon wants to insert the graft with the patient heparinized the intravenous heparin is given after blood has been taken for preclotting the graft. Heparinized blood cannot be used for preclotting.

Velour Grafts

Some grafts have a velour finish. A velour finish on the external surface is intended to help the graft embed in the surrounding tissues.

It is common for platelets to be deposited on the inner surface of fibre grafts and very occasionally clumps of platelets may be dislodged to give rise to an embolus. Some grafts are made with an inner velour surface so that any platelet thrombi will adhere more firmly, so making an embolus less likely.

Umbilical Vein Grafts

The umbilical vein graft was pioneered by Dardik and is sometimes known as the Dardik graft. It is used in cases where the long saphenous vein is not available for a graft distal to the inguinal ligament. The grafts are difficult to obtain and storage problems make them very expensive. They can cost more than £500 each.

Polytetrafluorethylene Grafts

These consist of expanded polytetrafluorethylene (PTFE) and are often called Gore-tex grafts. First described in 1972, they are used when the saphenous vein is indicated but not available. Reports concerning their success are variable.

Suture Materials

Over the years surgeons have used a great variety of suture materials and needles. Silk was initially used, and braided dacron has also been used more recently. Both these materials are braided. They may injure the artery wall, so making the suture hole bigger and they are sometimes difficult to pull through. Braided sutures such as silk have to be passed through liquid paraffin before being handed to the surgeon.

Many surgeons now use Prolene. This suture is monofilamentous and has the special quality of sliding very easily through the tissues. It does not need lubrication, and is very easy to use and causes minimal damage to the artery.

Needles

The size of needle used for arterial surgery varies according to the size of the artery. For aortic work a 25 mm needle is used, but for smaller arteries such as the femoral or popliteal artery a 10 mm or 13 mm needle is more convenient.

The strength of suture material is also different. For suturing the aorta 2/0 Prolene is used, but for the femoral or popliteal artery a 4/0 or 5/0 suture is more appropriate.

The needles used are round bodied or trocar pointed.

Suture Techniques

1. Interrupted sutures are commonly used when the surgeon is dealing with small arteries. This is because a small artery anastomosis may be narrowed when a continuous suture is pulled up.
2. For larger arteries and larger anastomoses a continuous suture technique is more usual. The surgeon usually passes a suture through each end of the anastomosis to make sure the two parts to be stitched are the same length, and then make a continuous suture.
3. It is sometimes convenient to use a double-ended suture. This is a suture with a needle at each end. One needle is passed through one corner of the anastomosis and the suture tied. Each needle is then carried up one side of the anastomosis and the two sutures are tied when they meet at the opposite corner. In this technique a single knot is used to complete the anastomosis.

5
The Sympathetic Nervous System

Anatomy of Spinal Nerves

The spinal cord runs within the spinal column. The spinal column comprises 24 individual bones or vertebrae from the skull to the lower lumbar region. This arrangement gives the spinal cord the protection which results from being within the bony canal, but as the spinal column is made up of 24 bones separated by discs of cartilage movement is possible. The spinal cord is shorter than the spinal column and ends at the lower end of the first lumbar vertebra in an adult.

Injury to the spinal cord is very serious but the surrounding spinal column gives good protection. All the motor nerves of the body begin in the brain and then run down in the spinal cord. At each segment of the body corresponding to a vertebra there is a spinal nerve which leaves the cord and emerges through a foramen between two vertebrae. This nerve leaves the cord towards the front and is called the anterior nerve root. It is then distributed to the muscles of the body, and impulses and messages concerning movement are sent via this route from the brain to the muscles.

All the sensory nerves of the body which bring sensations from the skin and other parts of the body collect together to join the large peripheral nerves. The motor and sensory nerves enter the spinal column through the intervertebral foramen. At this point they run together within a single nerve, but before entering the spinal cord the sensory nerves leave the motor nerves and run in a separate nerve root into the spinal cord. This is called the posterior nerve root which always has a ganglionated swelling on it.

The sensory nerves then ascend through the spinal cord to the brain where impulses are interpreted by the brain as subjective feelings.

Anatomy of Sympathetic Nerves

In addition to these motor and sensory nerves the sympathetic nerves pass through the spinal cord on their way to and from the brain and the periphery.

The sympathetic nerves carry impulses which are concerned with types of sensation and activity quite different from those of the ordinary spinal nerves. The sympathetic nerves supply the heart, lungs, and other viscera. They also supply the sweat glands and muscles controlling erection of the hairs of the skin and the muscle walls of the blood vessels.

The sympathetic nerves pass down the spinal cord from the brain in the same way as the ordinary motor nerves. However they do not leave the cord at every segment as do the spinal nerves. They leave in the anterior nerve roots from the first thoracic to the second lumbar nerves (Fig. 5.1).

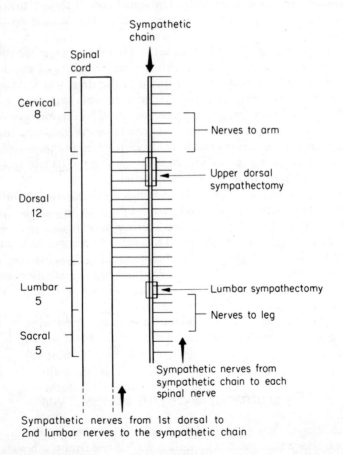

Fig. 5.1 The sympathetic nervous system.

The Sympathetic Chain

There are two sympathetic chains, one on each side of the body. In the neck the chain has three swellings or ganglia—the superior, middle, and inferior or stellate, and runs just behind the carotid artery. In the chest the chain runs under the pleura on the heads of the ribs where it can easily be seen through the pleura. In the lumbar region the chain runs on the front of the vertebral bodies. Throughout its length the sympathetic chain has ganglionated swellings.

The sympathetic nerves leave the spinal cord in the anterior nerve roots from the first thoracic to the second lumbar, and pass into the main spinal nerve root. The sympathetic nerves then leave the spinal root through a small communicating nerve to enter the sympathetic chain. The sympathetic nerves are finally distributed to the body in a variety of ways but the distribution to the limbs and blood vessels is through the peripheral nerves. Once in the sympathetic chain the nerve is relayed in a ganglion. It may then pass back to the spinal nerve at the same level through another communicating nerve. However, to reach all the peripheral nerves and so the whole body some sympathetic fibres will have to pass up and down the chain beyond the level of inflow (first thoracic to second lumbar) so that each spinal nerve in the body receives a communicating bunch from the sympathetic chain.

To summarize, the sympathetic nerves leave the cord from the first thoracic to the second lumbar nerves and enter the sympathetic chain. After relaying in ganglia the sympathetic nerves pass up and down the chain and then re-enter the spinal nerves through which they reach the peripheral arteries and other structures.

Physiology of Sympathetic Nervous System

The sympathetic nerves have many effects on the heart and other viscera. In this work we are only concerned with the effect on peripheral arteries. Any stimulation of the sympathetic system causes narrowing of the peripheral arteries and reduced blood supply, and division of the sympathetic nerves will cause dilatation of the arteries with consequent increase in blood flow and warmth. The sympathetic nerves also innervate the sweat glands so that after their division the skin of that part does not sweat. This can be an important check on completeness of sympathectomy. If a sympathectomy has been properly done the part should be warm and dry. If the skin still sweats then a sympathectomy has not been done.

Lumbar Sympathectomy

Indications

This operation is indicated when there is a need to increase the blood flow to the feet. In many patients with atherosclerosis the blood vessels are too rigid for any significant effect. Also it has no effect on the symptom of intermittent claudication as muscle flow is only marginally affected by the sympathetic system:

1. The main value of lumbar sympathectomy is in Buerger's disease. This is usually in younger men and the patient should be warned that when the operation is done on both sides there is a slight risk of impotence.
2. Some cases of atherosclerosis may receive sufficient benefit for the operation to be worthwhile. These are patients who have early rest pain or very early gangrene and are otherwise unsuitable for a grafting, reconstructive operation.

The Operation

The operation is not severe and both sides may be done at the same operation. The patient is placed flat on his back on the operating table. A horizontal incision about 10 cm long is made from the tip of the twelfth rib to 5–7 cm lateral to the umbilicus. The incision is deepened through the muscles of the abdominal wall but the membrane (peritoneum) which contains the intestines and other viscera is not incised, i.e., the approach is extraperitoneal. Instead it is separated from the muscle layer and pushed away from the back of the abdominal cavity. The sympathetic chain is picked up where it lies on the vertebral bodies and about 2 or 3 cm excised. This is usually about the level of lumbar two or three. The sympathetic nerves to the leg leave the spinal cord above the level of the second lumbar and at this point are passing down the chain before entering peripheral nerves lower down to reach the legs. There is some risk of damaging the inferior vena cava on the right side but damage to lumbar veins draining into the inferior vena cava is more likely to be the cause of troublesome bleeding.

Post-operative Observations

The patient's pulse and blood pressure should be recorded at 15-minute intervals. Retro-peritoneal haemorrhage is a rare complication which will cause elevation of the pulse rate and falling blood pressure.

It often takes some hours before the full effect of sympathectomy is noted in the feet.

Upper Dorsal Sympathectomy

Indications

This operation is used when a sympathectomy on the upper limb is required.

1. Raynaud's disease. Some cases of Raynaud's disease are very severe causing severe pain and gangrene of the fingers. Sympathectomy is very valuable in these cases but there is a tendency for the disease to recur after two or three years although it is never as severe.
2. Excessive perspiration (hyperhidrosis). It is obvious that this symptom should be incapacitating before an operation is advised but there are often compelling indications.
3. Other rare causes of finger ischaemia. These include Buerger's disease of the hand, cervical rib with thrombosis of the subclavian artery, and atherosclerotic occlusion of the subclavian artery.

The Operation

There are several routes to the upper dorsal (thoracic) chain but none are easy as the part of the chain which has to be removed lies on the heads of the first to fourth ribs and within the chest.

The cervical approach making an incision above the clavicle is still used by some surgeons but it is generally giving way to the more popular axillary approach.

Technique of Axillary Upper Dorsal Sympathectomy

Principle of the Operation

The sympathetic nerves to the arm leave the cord in the second to fourth or fifth thoracic nerves and enter the sympathetic chain through the communicating rami. They then pass up the chain and enter the nerves leading to the arm through communicating nerves. It is therefore sufficient to remove the chain from the level of the fourth rib to the second rib. It is preferable not to go higher as if the first dorsal ganglion or stellate ganglion (fusion of the last cervical and first dorsal ganglia) is damaged the sympathetic supply to the head will be damaged. This causes Horner's syndrome in which there is ptosis (dropping) of the eye lid, enophthalmos (sinking in of the eye ball—the opposite of exophthalmos), and a small pupil. Cosmetically this is undesirable, and particularly so if the operation is being performed on a young woman with Raynaud's disease.

The Operation

In a woman the incision is behind the breast. About 10 cm of the third rib is removed and rib-spreader used to separate the ribs. The lung is retracted and the chain is easily seen on the heads of the ribs and removed. The incision is deep and narrow, and a fibrelight cable is essential to give good illumination.

After removal of the chain the chest is closed. Drainage is not essential but if the surgeon does leave a drain in the chest it must be connected with an underwater seal.

Post-operative Observations

As this operation involves a thoracotomy a post-operative chest film is taken to ensure that the lung is fully expanded. The observations include 15-minute recording of the pulse and blood pressure. As the chest has been opened it is essential to observe the patient for cyanosis and shortness of breath which might indicate a collection of air or blood in the pleural cavity.

6
Arterial Embolism

Nearly all arterial emboli are thrombi detached from the wall of the heart and swept into the blood stream until they reach an arterial bifurcation where the vessel lumen is too small for the thrombus to pass any further. Once impacted the blood pounds the thrombus forcing it tightly into the lumen of the artery like a cork. This may result in complete ischaemia but usually some blood reaches the main artery beyond the embolus through collateral vessels and this may be sufficient to keep the part alive. Embolism is usually accompanied by spasm of the arterial tree resulting in severe pain and pallor of the limb. In the course of 4 to 6 hours the stagnant stream of blood distal to the embolus begins to coagulate and this is called a propagated thrombus (Fig. 1.2). To a lesser extent this also occurs above the embolus. If the ischaemia is complete the part will die and become infected with putrefying bacteria causing gangrene. In many other cases sufficient circulation is carried on through collateral vessels and the limb survives. If the collaterals are adequate and the patient is not very active he may not notice much wrong with the leg. However, in most cases of embolus which recover there is some reduction of blood flow to the limb and the patient will complain of intermittent claudication when he is able to walk again.

Sources of Arterial Emboli

1. The most common source of an embolus is the left atrium of the heart. Patients with mitral stenosis often develop atrial fibrillation, and in this condition when there are no normal contractions of the atrium thrombus is inclined to form inside the left atrium. Although it is usually attached to the wall of the heart fragments may become detached and form emboli. This often occurs in episodes, and a patient who has an embolus from the left atrium often gets several more unless effective treatment is instituted. An embolus often takes place when the rhythm of the heart is altered as for example when drugs or electrotherapy are used to convert fibrillation to normal rhythm. Embolus is also a dangerous

complication of the operation of closed mitral valvotomy when thrombus can be dislodged by the surgeon's index finger in the left atrium.

2. In some cases of coronary artery thrombosis the infarcted and necrotic heart muscle involves the lining of the wall of the ventricle, and thrombus forms on this necrotic endothelium (a mural thrombus). When the right ventricle is involved the thrombus may be detached and pass into the pulmonary artery causing a pulmonary embolus, and when the left ventricle is involved the thrombus may detach and pass into the aorta causing a systemic embolus. This complication is inclined to occur about 10 days after a coronary thrombosis. The patients in this group may have difficult cardiac problems and be much more difficult to handle surgically than those with atrial fibrillation complicating mitral stenosis.

3. Rarely thrombus forms on an ulcerated plaque of atheroma in the thoracic or abdominal aorta and this may also become detached to form a peripheral embolus.

4. *Paradoxical Embolus.* In this rare condition there is an atrial septal defect. A venous embolus reaches the right atrium and passes through the defect to the left atrium. It is now on the systemic side of the circulation and behaves as a systemic embolus.

Sites of Embolus

1. Lower Limbs

By far the most common part of the body to be affected by embolism is the lower limb. Emboli usually lodge at the aortic bifurcation (sometimes called saddle embolus), the division of the common iliac artery, the division of the common femoral artery into its superficial femoral and profunda branches or the division of the popliteal artery into its branches. An embolus at any of these sites gives rise to sudden and dramatic changes in the circulation in the leg. In addition to sudden pain caused by arterial spasm there will be colour changes and also the effects of ischaemia on various structures in the limb.

Clinical Picture of Embolism of the Arteries to the Leg

The colour change is usually a sudden pallor resulting from an emptying of blood from the limb. Sometimes the limb becomes a blotchy blue as a result of stagnation of blood in the limb. The oxygen is used from the blood resulting in the blue colour, and as the limb circulation is arrested the leg remains blue. The first tissues in the limb to feel the effects of severe ischaemia are the peripheral nerves which cease to function after about half an hour. The sensory nerves are unable to transmit impulses and the limb becomes anaesthetic. Lesser ischaemia may cause paraesthesiae such as tingling and 'pins and needles'. The inability of the motor nerves to transmit impulses causes paralysis of the muscles so that the patient is unable to move the limb. These signs of anaesthesia and paralysis are signs of serious ischaemia and indicate that the continued life of the limb is in peril unless the circulation can be restored. The muscles of the limb can withstand ischaemia for considerably longer. Total ischaemia can probably be tolerated for up to 8 hours. Death of muscle after this period is indicated by paralysis and by inflammatory changes in the skin overlying the muscle. Once this has happened and the main muscle mass is dead restoration of the circulation is useless.

There is no specific time which can be given as that in which the circulation must be restored if the limb is to survive. In some cases the collateral circulation is so good that a reasonable limb can be achieved without removal of the embolus, and there are varying degrees of competence of the collateral circulation which result in varying degrees of recovery. However, when surgical intervention is deferred more than 6 hours it becomes more difficult because of the formation of propagated clot which has to be dealt with in addition to the embolus before the circulation is restored (Fig. 1.2).

2. Upper Limb

Emboli in the arm are much less common than in the leg. There is another difference and this is that the collateral circulation in the arm is much richer than in the leg so that removal of the embolus is much less often required as the collateral circulation is sufficient to sustain the life of the arm.

Treatment of Arterial Emboli

The ischaemic leg should always be treated on the principles previously outlined.

NON-SURGICAL TREATMENT. As the patient has a cardiac pathology it is usually wise, particularly if the patient has had a recent coronary thrombosis, to call for the assistance of a cardiologist. Improvement in cardiac function may in itself help the circulation to the limb.

The main non-surgical treatment is anticoagulation with intravenous heparin. The object of anticoagulation is to prevent propagation of thrombosis which will obstruct collateral blood vessels and also present additional technical problems because the surgeon has to remove propagated thrombus in addition to the embolus. Heparin is the preferred anticoagulant as it is given intravenously and is immediately effective. Should an operation be required the heparin can be discontinued and it will be completely metabolized in 4 hours. Continuous heparin is given with an automatic clockwork syringe so that the patient can move about freely if he is able. The usual dose is 20 000 units every 12 hours, but the dose is regulated by doing the Thrombin Clotting Time (TCT). Full details of techniques of heparinization are given in Chapter 23.

SURGICAL TREATMENT. Should it be decided to remove the embolus the patient is prepared for the operating theatre. The operation may be performed under general or local anaesthetic, and if there is any serious anxiety about the heart local anaesthetic is preferred. An incision is made over the presumed site of the embolus and the surgeon exposes the artery. Usually it is necessary to identify an artery and its two branches, and these three arteries are controlled with small artery-controlling clamps (Bulldog clamps, Fig. 10.3). An incision is made into the artery and the embolus is removed. An important part of the operation is to ensure that no propagated clot is present. The proximal clamp can be momentarily removed to ensure that there is a good flow from above. Distal clearance is made with a Fogarty catheter (Fig. 6.1). This catheter has revolutionized the operation of embolectomy. It consists of a long plastic tube graduated in centimetres and with an inflatable balloon at its end. The catheter is inserted distally as far as possible and the balloon is then inflated with 0·5 to 2 ml of saline. The catheter is slowly withdrawn with the balloon inflated so that any clot is pulled out. Finally the arteriotomy is closed with arterial sutures. Most surgeons prefer to use three or four interrupted sutures for this.

Aortic Bifurcation Embolus (Saddle Embolus)

This operation used to be performed by approaching the bifurcation of the aorta through a long transperitoneal incision. The modern technique is to expose both femoral arteries in the thigh and to extract the clot from the aortic bifurcation using Fogarty catheters to pull out the clot. This operation can be performed under local anaesthetic and is now a relatively minor procedure (Fig. 6.1).

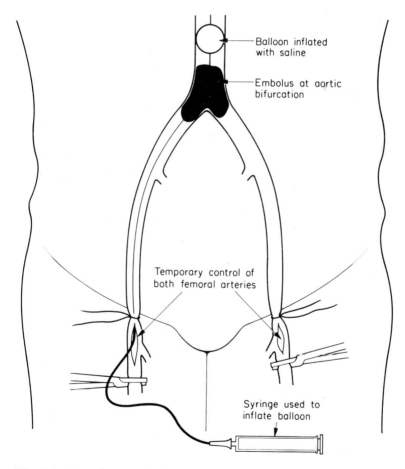

Balloon inflated
with saline

Embolus at aortic
bifurcation

Temporary control of
both femoral arteries

Syringe used to
inflate balloon

Fig. 6.1 Use of Fogarty balloon catheter to remove an aortic embolus. Both femoral arteries are controlled by clamps and the balloon catheter is passed up to bring the embolus down to the opening in the artery in the thigh.

OBSERVATIONS FOLLOWING THE OPERATION OF EMBOLECTOMY

1. Local observation of the wound. If there is leaking of blood from the arterial suture line a haematoma will form causing a swelling, or there may be bleeding from the incision.
2. If the thrombus has not been completely removed or if it recurs the limb will continue to show signs of ischaemia. It is important to watch the colour and temperature of the limb. In a successful case the limb colour and temperature rapidly returns to normal. If the limb does not return to normal appearance and temperature the surgeon should be informed before the patient leaves the recovery room.
3. Pulse volume recordings are invaluable in assessment of the success of the operation (page 17).

3. Cerebral circulation

Cerebral emboli are particularly serious and dramatic as when the embolus lodges in an end artery in the brain it causes cerebral ischaemia and the resulting brain damage causes a stroke of varying severity.

4. Mesenteric Embolism

When an embolus occludes the main superior mesenteric artery a very serious and dangerous state of affairs exists. There is no adequate collateral circulation and the small intestine becomes completely ischaemic. Unless the circulation can be restored within 6 hours the small intestine becomes gangrenous and the patient cannot survive.

The superior mesenteric artery supplies the whole of the small intestine and the ascending and transverse colon. When the origin of the artery from the aorta is occluded by an embolus the whole of this intestine becomes ischaemic. The patient is seized with severe and constant central abdominal pain. The proximal 30–45 cm of small intestine will receive some blood flow from anastomoses with the duodenal branches, and the colon may receive some nutrition via the marginal artery of the colon, so that most of the small bowel and some large intestine is completely ischaemic. As the bowel is infarcted blood is poured into its wall and into the lumen of the intestine causing the second important symptom of mesenteric embolism which is the passage of blood per rectum. At the same time the patient becomes shocked as a result of blood loss. Later the bowel organisms invade the dead intestine causing putrefying gangrene. These bacteria are often absorbed into the blood stream causing septicaemic shock. At this stage the patient has severe abdominal pain, and blood in the motions, and is in severe shock. The abdomen is distended and diffusely tender.

Treatment of Mesenteric Embolism

1. Until recently the only available treatment was resection of the gangrenous intestine. Unfortunately this is always an extensive resection, and even if the patient recovers there will be a severe problem of malnutrition because of inadequate absorption from the small length of intestine left after the resection.

2. *Embolectomy*. If the patient is diagnosed and explored before the onset of gangrene it may be possible to remove the embolus. This is done by putting an angled clamp on the aorta and then opening the artery over the embolus. After removal of the embolus the artery is closed with a few fine arterial sutures. In a successful case the colour immediately returns to the intestine.

7
Atherosclerosis: (1) General Description

Atherosclerosis, sometimes called arteriosclerosis or hardening of the arteries, is a disease of the arterial system. Although certain factors are known to make the disease worse the exact cause remains unknown. A normal artery is lined by a smooth layer of cells called the endothelium, or intima. In atherosclerosis yellow plaques appear on the arterial lining. These are particularly prominent at places where an artery branches. They are distributed throughout the body but are sometimes more prominent in one part of the body. However, when atherosclerosis is found in one place it is likely that the disease is widespread. Later the artery wall becomes thickened and may calcify. Many factors are known to predispose to atherosclerosis:

1. *Affluence*. Affluent societies are particularly liable to be troubled by atherosclerosis. Men who leave a poor country with a low incidence of atherosclerosis to live in a rich country become prone to the incidence of atherosclerosis of the country they have joined.

2. *Diet*. The people in poor countries tend to live on cereals. As they become richer and are able to grow more cereals they are able to use the surplus of cereals to feed and fatten animals. They then begin to take a diet with a high proportion of animal fat, and there is evidence that this is one factor in the cause of atherosclerosis.

3. *Hyperlipidaemia*. An elevated level of lipids in the blood stream carries a dangerous predisposition to atherosclerosis. In some cases this is familial, and subcutaneous deposits of lipids are seen in certain parts of the body. These are called xanthomas. Such patients have a very bad prognosis. Fatty acids are liberated into the blood stream by alcohol, and heavy drinking predisposes to atherosclerosis.

4. *Cigarette smoking*. There are now extensive data concerning the relationship of smoking with atherosclerosis. In particular the cigarette smoker is liable to early coronary thrombosis complicating atheroma in the coronary arteries and to arterial disease in the legs.

5. *Hypertension.* Patients with high blood pressure tend to early atherosclerosis, and effective treatment of the hypertension leaves the patient still liable to coronary thrombosis and other manifestations of atherosclerosis.

6. *Diabetes mellitus.* Clinicians have long known that diabetes predisposes to early atherosclerosis. Diabetic patients develop particularly bad atherosclerosis in the legs which is often difficult to treat surgically.

7. *Other factors.* Atherosclerosis is predominantly a disease of men. Obesity and stress are often cited as causative factors and patients with atherosclerosis are frequently overweight and employed in stressful occupations. However, there are no direct data to support this thesis, and it seems more likely that successful men develop the complications of atherosclerosis because of their eating and smoking habits.

Intimal Degeneration

As the plaque of atheroma grows it begins to cause turbulence of the blood flow and platelets from the blood are deposited on its surface. At this stage there is narrowing of the artery and some reduction of blood flow. When a stethoscope is placed over the narrow artery a systolic murmur may be heard as the blood rushes through the narrow part. Eventually the plaque so nearly occludes the lumen that the blood clots, causing a complete obstruction. The narrowing takes place over a period of months or years, and the body compensates for the reduced flow by creating alternative channels called collateral vessels (Fig. 1.1). The effectiveness of the collaterals is variable. In some cases it is so effective that the final thrombosis of the artery passes unnoticed. In others the collaterals do not develop well and thrombosis of the artery is accompanied by severe symptoms caused by the reduction of blood supply.

Calcification may appear in plaques of atheroma and this can be seen on plain radiographs. It may cause difficulty in a graft operation because of the difficulty of passing a suture through the calcified plaque.

Medial Degeneration

In some cases there is degeneration of the elastic and muscular media of the artery. The media is responsible for the elastic recoil of an artery. With each beat the blood is forced into the arteries which dilate to accommodate the blood. This is the mechanism of the pulse which can be felt at the wrist. When the heart rests after a contraction the muscle and elastic of the artery wall cause the artery to return to its former size. If the media is affected by atherosclerosis the muscle and elastic begin to degenerate and are less able to recoil after a heart beat. This causes an increase in the diameter of the arteries and a condition sometimes referred to as mega-arteries in which all the arteries of the body are dilated. In some cases the weakness is so great that the artery stretches much more to give rise to an aneurysm. The most common sites for this to happen are the abdominal aorta, the popliteal and the femoral artery.

8
Atherosclerosis: (2) Anatomy of the Circulation to the Lower Limbs

The abdominal aorta (Fig. 8.1) divides into two arteries called the common iliac arteries at a level which can be marked on the surface of

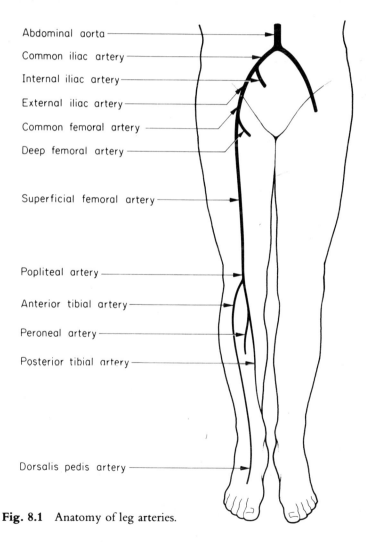

Fig. 8.1 Anatomy of leg arteries.

the body about 1–2 cm below and to the left of the umbilicus. Each common iliac artery is about 7–8 cm long and divides into an internal and external iliac artery. The internal iliac artery supplies the pelvic organs, the buttock (gluteal) muscles, and the external genital organs. The external iliac artery passes along the side of the pelvis to reach the thigh. It is relatively superficial when it reaches the thigh and its pulse should be sought just below the midpoint of the crease which marks the junction of the abdomen and the thigh.

In the thigh the main artery is called the common femoral artery. About 3 cm below the groin it gives off a branch called the deep branch of the femoral artery (profunda femoris) which supplies the thigh muscles. The main artery continues in a relatively superficial plane and is called the superficial femoral artery. It curves round the inner aspect of the thigh and close to the femur near its lower third to reach the back of the knee where it is called the popliteal artery. There are no large branches of the superficial femoral or the popliteal artery. Below the knee the popliteal artery divides into three arteries which are called the anterior tibial, posterior tibial, and peroneal arteries.

It is possible but difficult to feel the pulsation of the popliteal artery in the popliteal fossa behind the knee. In the middle of the dorsum of the foot it is possible to feel the pulse of the dorsalis pedis artery which is the continuation in the foot of the anterior tibial artery. The posterior tibial artery can normally be felt behind the bone on the inner aspect of the ankle (medial malleolus). The peroneal artery usually terminates deep in the leg and its pulse cannot be felt.

9
Atherosclerosis: (3) Aorto-Iliac Disease

Aorto-Iliac Disease

When there is narrowing or complete occlusion of the aorta the effects will be bilateral. Occlusion of the aorta and common iliac arteries gives rise to a reduction in blood flow in the internal and external iliac arteries. There is a free anastomosis in the pelvis between the two internal iliac arteries and this minimizes the effects.

1. *Intermittent claudication.* Because the blood flow to the leg is reduced claudication is frequently felt in the calf muscle. However, it is characteristic of aorto-iliac disease that claudication may be felt in the thigh or buttock.
2. *Gangrene.* This is an unusual feature of aorto-iliac disease because of the free anastomosis between the internal iliac arteries which carry sufficient blood to prevent gangrene. However, if there is a second occlusion in the superficial femoral or below gangrene may develop.
3. *Impotence.* A reduction of the blood flow to the internal iliac artery may result from disease in the aorta, common iliac or internal iliac artery. In addition to gluteal claudication the reduction of arterial flow to the penis may prevent erection. This combination of symptoms was described by Leriche and is now known as Leriche's syndrome.

Treatment of Aorto-Iliac Disease

The important principle is that the surgeon is dealing with very large arteries and reconstruction is relatively easy. The indications for surgery are:

1. Gangrene of the foot or toe. This is usually caused by a second occlusion in the thigh or lower, but reconstruction of the aorta or iliac artery will so improve the circulation that amputation will be avoided.
2. Intermittent claudication. This is always judged individually

but if the patient is seriously troubled and incapacitated then surgical treatment is indicated.

3. Impotence. Patients with this symptom rarely benefit from reconstructive surgery.

Dacron Graft

When the occlusion involves the common or external iliac arteries it may be bypassed with a 10 mm dacron tube. When the disease involves the aorta and one or both iliac arteries a bifurcation graft is used. This may be sutured end to end after resection of the aorta and iliac arteries. An alternative is to use a bifurcated graft as a bypass. The graft is taken from the front of the aorta to below the occlusion. Because of the large size of the blood vessels and of the graft late occlusion is rare. The pre- and post-operative treatment and observations are the same as for the operation for femoral artery recon-

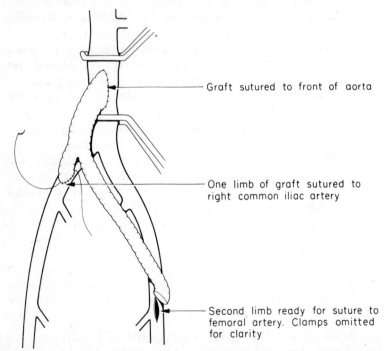

Graft sutured to front of aorta

One limb of graft sutured to right common iliac artery

Second limb ready for suture to femoral artery. Clamps omitted for clarity

Fig. 9.1   Dacron graft for aorto-iliac occlusion. The graft is shown sutured to the front of the aorta. The position of the distal suture lines is determined by the position of the occlusions. In this case the graft is being sutured to the right common iliac artery and to the left common femoral artery.

struction, and reference should be made to Chapter 10 for this information.

The aorta and iliac vessels may be approached in two ways.

1. TRANSPERITONEAL APPROACH. In this operation the inclusion is a vertical one in the centre of the abdomen. The peritoneal cavity is opened and the intestines are packed off and retracted to expose the great vessels which are at the back of the abdomen.

2. RETROPERITONEAL APPROACH. The abdominal incision is a curved one and is deepened down to, but not through, the peritoneal membrane. The peritoneum with its contained viscera and intestines is mobilized from the anterior and lateral, and finally from the posterior abdominal wall. It can be retracted to display the aorta and its main branches. This approach gives a much smoother convalescence but it is difficult in fat patients.

The rest of the operation is identical in both cases (Fig. 9.1). A woven graft is selected and pre-clotted. The patient is then fully heparinized by the anaesthetist. After clamping the aorta an opening is made in it and the graft sutured to the opening. A clamp is placed on the end of the graft and the aortic clamps are released. The arterial blood pressure within the graft causes it to lengthen, and after selection of a suitable place for the distal anastomosis the correct length is marked. The graft is then clamped more proximally, cut at the previously selected point, and anastomosed to the iliac or femoral artery.

Endarterectomy

This operation is variously named thrombo-endarterectomy, disobliteration, or reboring. It may be performed in two ways—open or closed.

1. OPEN ENDARTERECTOMY (Fig. 9.2). This is generally used for short occlusions such as the carotid or common iliac artery.

The affected artery is exposed by a suitable incision and fully mobilized so that clamps can be applied above and below the occluded area. The patient is heparinized before the clamps are applied. It is best to give the patient a full dose of intravenous heparin but some surgeons still prefer to inject heparin solution into the artery below the occlusion. This solution is made by adding 5000 units of heparin to 500 ml of saline.

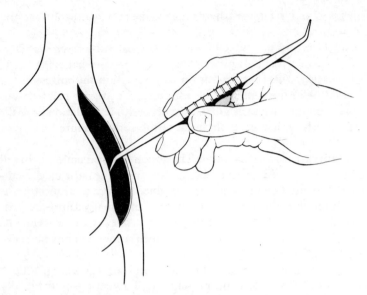

Fig. 9.2 Open endarterectomy using Watson–Cheyne dissector. The artery is of course clamped above and below to prevent bleeding. It is then incised and the occluding atheroma removed.

The surgeon then makes a longitudinal incision in the artery along the full length of the occlusion. The incision goes through the wall of the artery into the atheromatous part. The surgeon then seeks the plane of cleavage using the Watson–Cheyne dissector. Once in the correct plane the dissection proceeds until the whole plaque has been freed and can be removed.

In a large artery such as the iliac the incision is closed with a continuous prolene suture. In closing a small artery such as the carotid by this technique considerable narrowing would result so that it is better to close the incision with a vein patch to widen it.

2. CLOSED ENDARTERECTOMY is more suitable in smaller arteries and is described on page 53.

Observations following Reconstructive Operations on the Aorta and Iliac Arteries

1. The pulse and blood pressure are recorded at 15-minute intervals. Elevation of the pulse and fall in blood pressure may indicate bleeding from the suture lines. Sometimes

this may be shown by excessive bleeding into the suction drain.

2. The circulatory state of the legs is constantly observed. The patient is best nursed with the feet exposed so that colour and temperature changes can be observed. If a foot pulse can be felt its site is marked in ink so that it can be palpated at 15-minute intervals. Deterioration of the circulation or loss of the pulse may indicate thrombosis at the suture line, and the surgeon should be informed.

3. Urine output. Excessive haemorrhage is unusual in these operations but a period of hypotension during the operation may result in impaired renal function. It is usual to have a catheter in the bladder so that the renal output can be measured, and it should be at least 1·5 ml per minute.

4. When the operation is transperitoneal there will be temporary paralytic ileus. A Ryles tube (intragastric tube) is left in the stomach and the hourly aspirate is measured.

10
Atherosclerosis: (4)
Femoro–Popliteal Disease

Atherosclerotic narrowing and occlusion in this area usually begins at the junction of the femoral and popliteal arteries which is about the junction of the middle and lower thirds of the thigh. Once a complete occlusion has taken place the column of blood above it has virtually no flow; and so it thromboses. The extent of this thrombosis is variable. There may be a short occlusion some 5 cm in length, or the occlusion may extend proximally to the origin of the profunda femoris artery.

The proximal part of the popliteal artery is also affected at times, but the distal part of the popliteal artery usually remains patent and relatively free from atherosclerosis.

A third important site of atheroma is at the origin of the profunda femoris artery which may be considerably narrowed by athero-sclerosis. This is important because when the superficial femoral artery is occluded a limited flow reaches the patent arteries below the obstruction through collateral branches which are derived from the profunda femoris artery.

Intermittent Claudication

The characteristic feature of femoro–popliteal occlusion is intermit-tent claudication which is felt in the calf of the leg. Some patients who are elderly and retired may be able to live with this symptom. In others the symptom is severely incapacitating and may prevent the patient from working or from getting to his work. In these patients surgical treatment has to be considered after careful assessment of the rest of the cardiovascular system. In some patients with coronary atherosclerosis causing angina it may be very unwise to operate on the leg to enable the patient to walk faster and further because this will have the effect of making his cardiac condition worse and may cause a fatal attack of coronary insufficiency.

Gangrene

When gangrene and rest pain are present an attempt to reconstruct the occluded artery should always be made. The alternative is an amputation and this is an operation of equal severity and, of course, the post-operative treatment and convalescence is so much more difficult after an amputation. Following a successful graft operation a limited area of toe gangrene will separate. If gangrene is more extensive a local amputation will be necessary.

Amputation

When reconstructive surgery is technically impossible a major amputation is usually inevitable.

Treatment of Femoro-Popliteal Occlusions

Medical Treatment

This is indicated when claudication is mild and not interfering with the patient's way of life or his ability to earn his living. The important aspects of medical treatment are:

1. It is essential that the patient stops smoking cigarettes.
2. Exercise may contribute to the formation of a collateral circulation, and the patient should be encouraged to walk as much as he is able.
3. Correction of blood abnormalities. It is obvious that any degree of anaemia should be corrected as the oxygen-carrying capacity of the blood is reduced in anaemia. Correction of anaemia may improve intermittent claudication.

   Polycythaemia is a condition in which the number of red cells is increased and the haemoglobin elevated. This condition causes an increase in the viscosity of the blood, and its correction by medical means will enable blood to flow through the legs more easily and so alleviate intermittent claudication.
4. Vasodilator drugs. A great number of vasodilator drugs have been marketed in recent years. Although they are frequently prescribed there is no real evidence that they benefit a patient with calf claudication due to a femoro-popliteal artery

occlusion. The drugs are given orally and have a generalized vasodilator effect. This may cause blood to be diverted to other parts of the body so that the limb with an obstructed artery gets even less blood. There is also a tendency for the blood pressure to fall and the heart has to work harder to maintain the blood pressure and perfusion through an increased volume of vascular system. Many of these patients have coronary artery disease and may develop angina as a result of the increase of work done by the heart.

5. Anticoagulant drugs have not been effective in arresting the progress of this disease.

Surgical Treatment

1. Intermittent Claudication

Surgical treatment may be indicated in a patient with intermittent claudication if it is sufficiently severe to interfere with his enjoyment of life or his ability to work. However, it must be judged against the background of the generalized nature of the disease. Treatment is usually only advised when one leg is involved and there is no evidence of marked disease in other parts of the body.

2. Gangrene and Rest Pain

When the patient is threatened with a major amputation because of rest pain and gangrene it is always worth trying to do some form of operation which will restore the blood flow and avoid an amputation. It is quite justifiable to operate on poor risk cases with evidence of generalized atherosclerosis.

Clinical Examination and Investigations

The patient is examined to determine the extent of the disease. Investigations are also made of other manifestations of the disease as well as an exact anatomical diagnosis of the occlusion in the leg.

URINE. Diabetes mellitus is a common complication, and routine examination of the urine for sugar and ketones is mandatory.

CARDIOVASCULAR EXAMINATION. In addition to the usual examination of the heart the common sites of atherosclerosis are examined. The abdomen should be examined for aneurysm, and the neck for carotid stenosis.

An ECG should be done to determine the presence of significant interference with the blood supply to the heart resulting from atheromatous plaques causing narrowing of the coronary arteries.

PULMONARY EXAMINATION. Many patients with atherosclerosis have been heavy smokers, and examination of the chest will often show evidence of bronchitis and emphysema. A radiograph of the chest will also be taken.

ARTERIOGRAPHY. The exact anatomical site of the occlusion can only be determined by arteriography which is fully described in Chapter 3. An operation cannot be performed without good arteriographic studies.

Preparation for Surgery

Most patients who need surgical treatment for atherosclerosis will need 5 or 6 days' treatment to improve the function of the lungs. The patient must not be confined to bed as this will result in poor breathing and possible collapse of segments of lung. In addition to active mobilization he will need the assistance of the physiotherapist with breathing exercises. Should active bronchitis be present it may be wise to give a short course of antibiotics.

Most surgeons use a cover of prophylactic antibiotics as infection of a wound following artery operation carries a serious risk of fatal secondary haemorrhage. A broad spectrum antibiotic is started on the day before the operation.

Skin preparation for an operation on the femoral or popliteal artery is often a major undertaking. Frequent bathing is necessary with particular attention to the groin which should be powdered after bathing with an antiseptic powder. The shaving will need to be from the nipples, to include the whole abdomen and pubis, going down to midcalf on the side of the operation.

Operations for Femoro–Popliteal Occlusion

1. LUMBAR SYMPATHECTOMY. This operation is still sometimes performed for patients with very minor degrees of necrosis in the toes or rest pain. It is valueless for intermittent claudication. Sometimes the sympathetic chain may be destroyed by an injection of phenol. The operation of lumbar sympathectomy is described in Chapter 5.

2. ARTERIAL RECONSTRUCTION. Three techniques are available for arterial reconstruction of the femoral or popliteal arteries.

1. The most usually performed and most successful operation is the use of the long saphenous vein. This vein possesses valves which only allow the flow of blood towards the heart. It is therefore necessary to remove the vein and to reverse its direction before inserting it into the artery. The vein must be at least 4 mm in diameter if a successful result is to be achieved.
2. ENDARTERECTOMY. This operation leaves the inside of the artery without an intimal lining and is generally unsuccessful in arteries of this size though it may be successful in larger arteries.
3. Thirdly the surgeon may use another form of tube. The umbilical vein graft is most likely to be successful but is very expensive. Dacron or Gore-tex tubes are also used but longer term reports have not been very favourable. These techniques are only used when there is no suitable saphenous vein.

Technique of Long Saphenous Vein Graft

The patient is given a general anaesthetic and the diathermy electrode placed on the opposite leg. Sometimes, particularly in women, a catheter is left in the bladder for a few days.

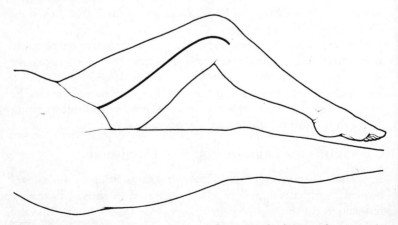

Fig. 10.1 Position of patient and site of incision for long saphenous vein graft.

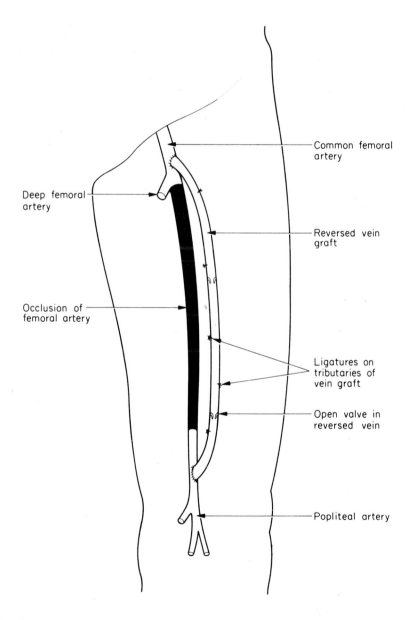

Fig. 10.2 Long saphenous bypass graft to femoral artery.

The femoral artery runs from the mid-point of the groin and down the inner aspect of the thigh. The popliteal artery lies behind the knee but is approached via an incision along the inner aspect of the knee. To gain access to the whole of this it is necessary to pay special attention to the position of the patient on the table. A small cushion is placed under the opposite buttock, and it is useful to have a table with a lateral tilt to increase the angle when the surgeon is working on the inner aspect of the knee. The hip and knee are both flexed about 20° and the position of the foot secured with two sand bags (Figs. 10.1, 10.2).

After towelling the surgeon exposes the long saphenous vein. This may be done through a number of small transverse incisions or a long incision over it. The branches are ligated and divided, and when a sufficient length has been secured it is removed and taken to a separate table. Here it is inflated with saline, and any holes or un-ligated branches are tied.

The surgeon then turns to the artery and exposes it above and below the sites of the occlusion. Once all is ready for insertion of the graft the patient is heparinized with an intravenous injection of heparin. The dose is 100 units to 1 kilogram of body weight so that a 70 kilogram man will receive 7000 units of heparin. Some surgeons use local heparin prepared by adding 1000 units of heparin to 100 ml of saline. This solution is injected into the artery below the clamp.

The artery is now controlled by the application of atraugrip clamps or Bulldog clips (Fig. 10.3) and opened with a fine scalpel. The surgeon may wish to use Potts scissors (Fig. 10.4) for this part of the operation. The vein graft is then sutured to the openings in the artery taking care that its direction is reversed. It is usual to use small needles of about 12–15 mm length and fine suture material of about 5/0 size for these anastomoses (Fig. 10.2).

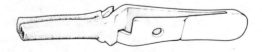

Fig. 10.3 Small cross-action artery clamp for control of medium-sized arteries. It is usually called a Bulldog clamp. The small hole in the handle is for a suture as these small instruments have been left in a wound. They should always be counted like sponges.

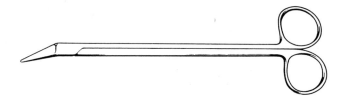

Fig. 10.4 Potts scissors. These pointed and angled scissors are used to open a blood vessel.

After completion of the anastomosis and closure of the wounds the surgeon will generally need one or two suction drains. These drains are secured with sutures.

Closed Endarterectomy (Fig. 10.5)

The patient is anaesthetized and the area towelled to give access to the artery at each end of the occlusion. The artery is exposed above and below the occlusion through separate incisions. The patient is heparinized and, after clamping, the artery is incised longitudinally for about 2 cm at the lower end of the occlusion, partly over it and partly over patent artery below. The Watson–Cheyne dissector is used to dissect out the core which is to be disobliterated, and when about 1 cm has been freed a loop endarterectomy stripper is passed over it. The stripper is then gently passed proximally until it reaches the proximal end of the occlusion where the artery is opened and the core broken off and removed.

This operation is easy to describe but not always easy to do. Also there is a high incidence of early failure due to thrombosis of the endarterectomized segment.

Profundoplasty

When there is no possibility of doing a graft of any kind this operation is sometimes done. The principle is that when the main superficial femoral artery is occluded the circulation through the collaterals may be improved by widening the upper part of the deep (Profunda) branch of the common femoral artery.

The patient is prepared in a similar way to the long saphenous vein graft operation. He is placed flat on the table and an incision made in the proximal part of the thigh over the femoral artery. The main

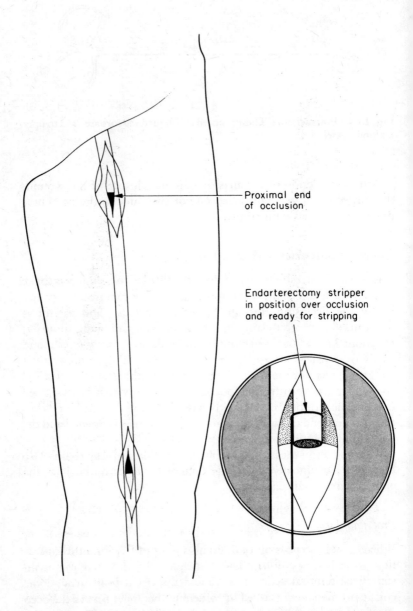

Proximal end
of occlusion

Endarterectomy stripper
in position over occlusion
and ready for stripping

Fig. 10.5 Closed endarterectomy. In this case the femoral artery has been exposed in two places corresponding with the upper and lower limits of the occlusion. The occluding segment has been freed below and the stripper engaged.

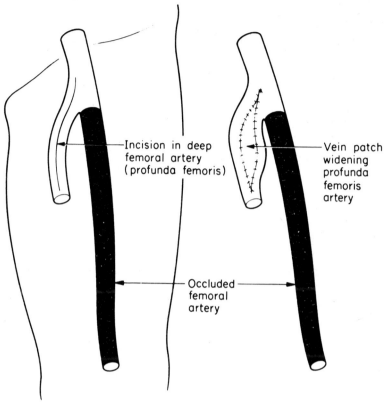

Incision in deep
femoral artery
(profunda femoris)

Vein patch
widening
profunda
femoris
artery

Occluded
femoral
artery

Fig. 10.6 Profundoplasty. An incision is made in the deep femoral artery
which is then widened with a vein patch.

artery and its profunda branch are exposed, and the entrance to the
profunda is widened by making an incision in it and repairing it with
a patch from the saphenous vein (Fig. 10.6).

Post-operative Management and Observations

1. In the recovery room and for some hours it is necessary to
   watch the patient for haemorrhage from the suture lines.
   This will be diagnosed by observation of the leg and the
   drain. Excessive loss of blood from the Redivac drain or
   swelling indicating haematoma should be reported to the
   surgeon at once, and it is occasionally necessary for a patient
   to be returned to theatre for bleeding to be stopped. The
   pulse and blood pressure are recorded every 15 minutes.
2. The patient should be watched carefully for early closure of

the graft which is also an indication for the patient to be returned to theatre. It is essential to nurse the patient with a cradle over the feet and the feet exposed. Any sudden change in colour should be reported at once. Following a successful operation the foot should be warm and pink. It is usually warmer than its fellow and it should become increasingly warm in the first 24 hours after the operation. Any sudden cooling should be reported to the surgeon at once. Sometimes it is possible to feel the foot pulses and if this is so it is an easy matter to observe them at hourly intervals. The use of pulse volume recordings is essential to establish the success of the operation. Clinical observations are sometimes difficult to interpret.

The patient may be allowed to walk in 48 hours, and the suction draining removed when daily drainage is less than 5 ml. Some surgeons immobilize the knee joint for 4 or 5 days particularly if the distal anastomosis is below the knee joint and may be placed under tension when the knee joint is moved.

11
Amputations

Amputation is called for in vascular disease or trauma when the effects of the lack of blood are very severe and surgical treatment to restore the blood supply is impossible. Most amputations for vascular disease involve the lower extremity.

Indications for Amputation in Vascular Disease

1. GANGRENE AND REST PAIN. Severe reduction in blood supply (ischaemia) causes death of the tissue which then becomes infected. This dead tissue is called gangrene and usually begins in a toe but is inclined to spread to the foot. Gangrene is usually a very painful condition preventing sleep at night and rest in the day. The patient may require strong narcotic drugs for the relief of pain which may be so intolerable that he asks for amputation. This symptom is called rest pain and is occasionally present before the onset of gangrene.

2. INFECTION. In some cases of gangrene the dead tissue is invaded by virulent bacteria and this infection spreads to the rest of the leg causing serious illness. Severe spreading infection is sometimes an indication for amputation. This is particularly common in diabetic patients.

3. MASSIVE NECROSIS OF MUSCLE. When there is sudden ischaemia the large muscle bellies may become ischaemic and die. The absorption of the products of dead muscle are very toxic to the patient who may become extremely ill. Amputation in such a case results in dramatic improvement within a few hours.

Principles of Amputation

Psychological Help

Many elderly patients are very distressed when told that major amputation is necessary. Although some will obviously not walk again it is important to help and encourage as much as possible. If

there is a patient available who has had an amputation and who is
well rehabilitated and walking, he should be asked to visit the patient
before his operation. The sight of a fellow sufferer who is walking
again will give confidence and act as a real stimulus to get better and
not to give up.

Myoplastic Amputation

There is no place for the old amputation in which bone and muscle
were divided at the same level. The object was to create a cone-
shaped stump by retraction of muscle from the stump in which the
bone end was covered by skin. Daily bandaging of the stump was
carried out after the amputation to assist the production of the
cone-shaped stump. The fitter made an appliance which contained
the limb with the stump hanging loosely inside, and all the weight
was taken through the artificial limb to the tuberosity of the ischium
in the buttock. Such a small weight-bearing area caused pain and
instability on walking.

No tourniquet is necessary in amputation for gangrene as bleeding
will not be excessive. It is also possible to damage an atherosclerotic
artery because it is rigid and inelastic. Whereas a normal elastic artery
is compressed and occluded by a tourniquet a rigid artery may be
fractured and permanently occluded.

The construction of the flaps varies with different amputations
and is based on the knowledge of the blood supply to the flap.

With the exception of knee joint and Stokes Gritti amputation the
modern amputation is performed as a myoplastic operation. This
means that the muscles are carefully divided so that they can be used
to cover the cut end of the bone. It is the intention to make an
appliance which snugly fits the stump, so spreading the weight over
a wide area of contact and then through the patient's own joints.

Level of Amputation

The surgeon takes many factors into account when judging the level
of amputation.

When the arterial occlusion is distal a conservative amputation of a
gangrenous toe is indicated.

When a gangrenous toe is caused by extensive atherosclerotic
occlusion of the femoral and popliteal artery a major proximal
amputation is inevitable. The thigh receives a good blood supply
from the deep branch of the femoral artery, but amputation of the toe

or foot will be followed by failure to heal and recurrent gangrene. It is often difficult to explain to a patient with gangrene of the toe that he needs an amputation around the level of the knee joint.

It is important in elderly patients to preserve as much leg as possible, and in some cases the surgeon will be able to do an amputation 4 or 5 inches below the knee. More often he will have to advise an amputation at about knee joint level.

Above-knee Myoplastic Amputation (Fig. 11.1)

In this operation the femur is divided about 7 inches above the knee joint. The thigh muscles are cut at a lower level giving sufficient length to suture them over the cut end of the bone. The equal anterior and posterior skin flaps are sutured accurately. Most amputations are closed with a suction (Redivac) drain. Of all amputations for gangrene this one has the highest mortality.

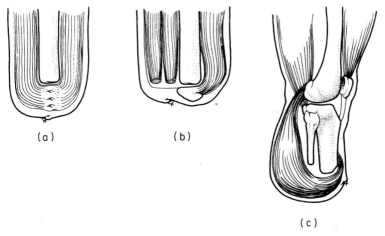

(a) (b) (c)

Fig. 11.1 (a) Myoplastic amputation of thigh. Note muscles sutured over bone end. (b) Stokes–Gritti amputation. The patella is placed over the cut end of the femur. (c) Below-knee amputation. The calf muscle is sutured over the bone end. The fibula is cut shorter and the tibia bevelled in front.

Amputation through the Knee Joint

Skin flaps are cut below the knee joint. The leg is severed through the knee joint by cutting the collateral ligaments on each side of the joint and the strong cruciate ligaments which hold the femur to the tibia. The section is entirely through the joint and no bone is divided. The patella ligament is sutured to the stump of the cruciate ligaments to prevent muscle retraction. The large area of bone allows end weight-bearing on this stump.

Supracondylar Amputation—Stokes Gritti

This is a very popular amputation among vascular surgeons. The anterior flap comes just below the patella and is carried deeply so that it contains the patella. The femur is divided just above its condyle and the articular part of the patella is removed with a saw. When the anterior flap is put in position over the stump the patella lies in contact with the end of the femur, and bony union should take place. Fixation is unnecessary.

This operation is popular among surgeons as it carries a very high rate of healing. It is unfortunate that the patella is only about 5 square centimetres as this is too small an area for end weightbearing.

Below-knee Amputation

There are several techniques for performing this amputation. The amputation is most conveniently done with the patient lying on his back. The anterior incision is made half way round the leg at the site of bone section. The posterior flap is long and contains the gastrocnemius muscle. To avoid damage the bone section is conveniently done with a wire saw (Gigli) and the posterior flap containing muscle covers the bone end.

The presence of a normal knee joint is the great advantage of this operation.

Symes Amputation

This operation is not usually indicated for vascular disease as it is too distal and healing will not take place. However, if a successful graft operation has been done for gangrene of the toes extending to the foot a Symes amputation will give a very satisfactory result.

In the Symes amputation the skin of the heel forms the flap and it is cut from the heel bone (os calcis). An incision is also made across the front of the ankle and the tibia divided just above its articular surface. The heel flap is then sutured over the cut end of the bone. One advantage of this operation is that the patient can walk about on a carpet at home without any form of artificial limb. When fitted with a prosthesis the skin is strong enough for the patient's full weight to be borne on its end.

Limb Fitting and Convalescence

The limb fitter will provide the artificial limb. The only part which is individually constructed is the socket which fits exactly the contour of the limb. This is called a total bearing socket. It may take some months before the limb reaches its final size and shape so that the final limb may not be fitted for about three months. The below-knee prosthesis takes some weight on the patella tendon and is called a patella tendon prosthesis (PTB).

While waiting for the final fitted artificial limb the patient is given a simple appliance called a pylon. He is able to walk on this and get confidence while waiting for the limb to stabilize in shape for fitting and manufacture of the permanent limb. During this period the patient needs strong support particularly from those who have recovered from amputations and returned to normal life. Some of the workers in limb-fitting centres have had amputations.

Late Problems

The Home Nurse may encounter problems in amputees. The painful stump is the most common difficulty and, if troublesome, the patient should be referred to the limb fitter. In some cases a sore place develops because of movement, and some modification of the socket may be indicated. In other cases there is something wrong with the stump. There may be incomplete healing or a stitch sinus requiring surgery.

The main cut nerve stump may grow out forming a painful lump of nerve fibres called a neuroma. If this is near the scar it may be necessary to excise more nerve to allow the end to lie higher in the thigh where it is protected by the thigh muscles.

The Home Nurse should also watch the remaining limb. Many cases develop similar trouble on the second leg, and timely consultation may enable the surgeon to do a reconstructive artery operation and so avoid the tragedy of a second amputation.

Patients often complain that they feel the limb and move the toes although it has been amputated. This is called phantom limb, and is usually permanent. The feelings come from the part of the brain which previously interpreted sensations from the limb. Sometimes the phantom limb is painful. This is called causalgia. Luckily it rarely persists more than a few weeks after amputation.

12
Aneurysms

False Aneurysm

An aneurysm may be true or false. A true aneurysm is a dilatation or swelling of an artery. A false aneurysm which is also described in Chapter 19, is so called because it has the outward appearance and signs of a swollen, dilated artery. In fact a false aneurysm always results from an accident to an artery. Blood escapes from the damaged artery and forms a collection (a haematoma) adjacent to the artery. Because of the pulsation of the arterial blood such a collection of blood forms a pulsating swelling indistinguishable from a swelling of the artery itself. False aneurysms often occur on the limbs where an artery is damaged in an accident or as a result of a knifing incident.

Treatment of False Aneurysm

When an aneurysm is present in a limb it is safer to do the operation under a tourniquet.

Resection of the Aneurysm

If the hole in the artery is large it may be necessary to remove the short length of injured artery and to replace it with a vein graft. In the limbs the main artery is always accompanied by veins and an important nerve. These structures are liable to accidental damage when a false aneurysm is removed.

Aneurysm Repair

Because of the risk of damage to the main veins and nerves it is often possible to repair the artery by making an incision into the aneurysm. The operation is done under a tourniquet, and blood and clot removed from the sac. The defect in the artery is seen at the bottom of the false aneurysm sac and can easily be repaired with some interrupted arterial sutures. The cavity is drained with a suction drain and the wound closed.

True Aneurysm

There are many causes of aneurysms but all are concerned with some disease process in the wall of the artery which weakens it and causes it to swell or dilate under the pressure.

Atherosclerotic Aneurysm

Most aneurysms seen at the present time are the result of atherosclerotic degeneration. The most common site is the abdominal aorta below the renal arteries, but aneurysms may occur at any place, particularly in the femoral and popliteal arteries.

Congenital Aneurysm

Congenital aneurysm is rare except in the skull where aneurysms are sometimes present on the arteries which make up the circle of Willis (Fig. 15.1). These aneurysms may rupture, causing bleeding into the brain, which is damaged as a result.

Infective Aneurysms

In the condition known as bacterial endocarditis small infected thrombi are present on the heart valves. Although this condition can now be successfully treated with antibiotics small fragments of infected thrombus may occasionally be swept off in the blood stream, and these tiny pieces are arrested in a small peripheral artery. Here the bacteria invade the wall of the artery and weaken it, causing an aneurysm. This particular type of aneurysm is called a mycotic aneurysm.

The other infection which affects arteries causing aneurysm is syphilis. This particularly affects the arch of the aorta in the chest. Infective aneurysms are now very rare.

Anatomical Types of Aneurysm

Most aneurysms are fusiform in shape and are called fusiform aneurysms. When the weakness is more localized, as happens in syphilis, the aneurysm is likely to be on one aspect of the artery and this is called a saccular aneurysm.

Abdominal Aortic Aneurysm

These aneurysms are the most commonly seen at the present time and are the result of atherosclerotic degeneration weakening the wall of the aorta. They may affect the whole aorta but are often confined to the abdominal aorta below the renal arteries.

Another rare cause of aortic aneurysm is the congenital disease known as Marfan's Syndrome. This syndrome is characterized by the fact that the patient has long arms and fingers (arachnodactyly or spider fingers) and a congenital weakness of the media of the arteries. This weakness gives rise to the possibility of multiple aneurysms.

CLINICAL PRESENTATION OF AORTIC ANEURYSM. Most patients with atherosclerosis are ageing and are usually men in the age group above 60 years. As people are living longer the condition is becoming more common.

RUPTURE. Sometimes the first sign of an aortic aneurysm is rupture (Fig. 12.1). If the aneurysm ruptures into the peritoneal cavity the patient will bleed to death in a few minutes and will not survive long enough to reach hospital. More often the aneurysm ruptures retroperitoneally. The blood is confined by the peritoneum and clots

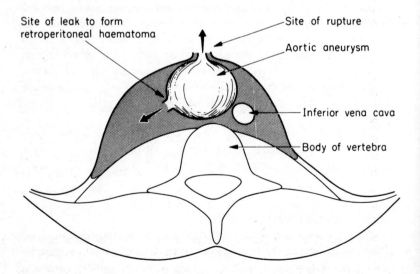

Site of leak to form
retroperitoneal haematoma

Site of rupture

Aortic aneurysm

Inferior vena cava

Body of vertebra

Fig. 12.1 Leaking aortic aneurysm.

retroperitoneally. The patient will suffer from the effects of a large retroperitoneal haematoma but the bleeding usually stops. This course of events is more properly referred to as a leaking aneurysm. Once an aneurysm has leaked recurrence and fatal haemorrhage is inevitable. However, the surgeon has time and opportunity to repair the damaged aorta.

The signs of leaking aneurysm are twofold.

1. The patient shows all the signs of acute bleeding; i.e., he is admitted to hospital in a state of shock with a rapid pulse, low blood pressure, sweating and pallor of the skin.
2. There are symptoms and signs referable to the aneurysm. The retroperitoneal haematoma causes pain in the back which is often severe. Some blood may leak into the peritoneal cavity where it irritates the peritoneum and causes pain and tenderness in the abdomen. When the surgeon examines the abdomen the pulsating aneurysm is easily felt.

TREATMENT OF LEAKING AORTIC ANEURYSM. Once an aneurysm is leaking the patient's only hope of survival is an operation to stop the bleeding. This comprises resection of the aneurysm and the insertion of a dacron graft to re-establish the aortic blood flow (Fig. 12.2). Often the patient is a poor risk because of cardiac and other manifestations of atherosclerosis in addition to shock resulting from haemorrhage, so that the mortality of this operation is in the region of 40% in good hands.

PULSATING MASS IN THE ABDOMEN. Many cases of aortic aneurysm are entirely symptomless and may be diagnosed by a physician making a routine examination.

Sometimes the patient will be aware of a pulsating mass in the abdominal cavity. Some patients do not feel the mass but are aware of the pulsation and say that they can feel their heart beating in the abdomen. The aneurysm may remain static in size for a long time but in other cases it may enlarge and rupture. Aneurysms more than 7 cm in diameter and those which are obviously getting bigger are dangerous because of the likelihood of rupture. Pain in the back is also a dangerous symptom.

Many patients are dead within a year following diagnosis of abdominal aortic aneurysm. However, most of the deaths are due to other manifestations of atherosclerosis which is usually severe in these cases. Patients die of heart failure, coronary thrombosis, and

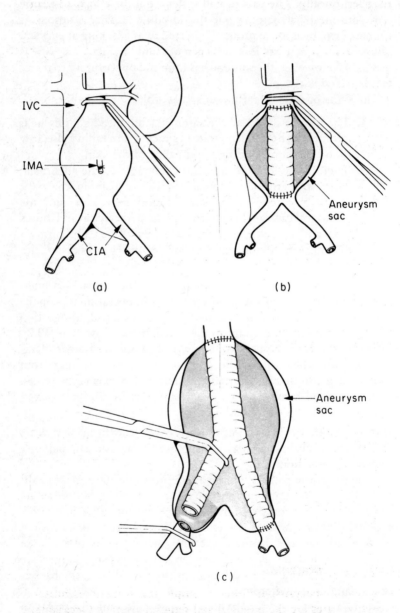

Fig. 12.2 (a) Aortic aneurysm; proximal clamp. LRV, left renal vein; IVC, inferior vena cava; IMA, inferior mesenteric artery (ligated); CIA, common iliac arteries. (b) Inlay Dacron tube graft. (c) Bifurcated Dacron graft.

strokes (cerebral haemorrhage). Of course some patients die as a result of rupture or leakage from the aneurysm, and this possibility is the only indication for advising surgical treatment for an unruptured aneurysm.

TREATMENT OF UNCOMPLICATED ANEURYSM OF THE ABDOMINAL AORTA. The modern treatment comprises resection of the aneurysm and the insertion of a dacron graft. However, the operation should only be advised in patients who are reasonably fit. Some are suffering from other and severe manifestations of generalized atherosclerosis. Also the operation need not be advised for a small aneurysm which is not enlarging nor causing back pain. The surgeon must take these factors into account when advising surgical treatment.

An alternative treatment which is much simpler and safer is to insert a length of wire into the aneurysm to induce clotting and so reduce the risk of rupture. This treatment is now rarely performed as there is little evidence that rupture is prevented.

Laboratory Studies

Radiographs taken in the antero-posterior and lateral positions usually confirm the presence of an aneurysm, and the outline is often marked by patchy calcification in the wall of the aneurysm. In doubtful cases the diagnosis can be confirmed and the diameter measured by ultrasonic studies.

Aortography is rarely performed. The aneurysm is partly filled with laminated clot and the lumen may be difficult to find. In addition there is a risk that the aortography needle might dislodge fragments of thrombus which would pass into and block the arteries of the legs.

Peripheral Aneurysms

Peripheral aneurysms are often multiple and sometimes bilateral. Common sites are the popliteal and femoral arteries. Occasionally they occur in the carotid or subclavian arteries. The pathology is atherosclerosis, and in some cases there is an associated aneurysm of the abdominal aorta.

Popliteal Artery Aneurysm

This occurs in elderly men and is often bilateral.

Some cases are benign and follow an uncomplicated course for many years. However, there is always great danger to the leg which may result from complete thrombosis of the aneurysm or from the detachment of small fragments of thrombus into the leg arteries. Complete occlusion of the popliteal artery or of the arteries below the knee causes gangrene and usually results in a major amputation.

Rupture of an aneurysm of the popliteal artery is a less common complication. As the artery is deeply placed in soft tissue haemorrhage causes swelling and bruising, but fatal loss of blood is impossible.

TREATMENT OF POPLITEAL ANEURYSM. Thrombosis and embolization are likely to come without warning so that provided the patient's general condition is reasonable an operation is indicated while the aneurysm is quiescent and patent.

The popliteal artery is reached by an incision down the back or medial side of the knee. After giving heparin and clamping the artery, the aneurysm is excised and any defect repaired with a reversed saphenous vein graft.

Femoral Artery Aneurysm

Like popliteal aneurysm this is also always atherosclerotic in origin. Also rupture is rare, and the sudden onset of ischaemia is due to thrombosis of the aneurysm or the detachment of small fragments of thrombus causing blockage of the arteries lower in the leg.

If the patient's condition permits, these aneurysms should be treated by excision followed by a graft using the saphenous vein. The operation is similar to that on the popliteal aneurysm but easier because access is less difficult.

13
The Operation of Excision of Abdominal Aortic Aneurysm

The operation does not differ in cases of uncomplicated and of leaking aneurysm but the pre- and post-operative treatment is more complicated in the cases which are leaking and the mortality is higher.

Prevention of Renal Failure

This serious complication can largely be eliminated by adopting measures which will keep the patient's urine flow high. Blood loss must be replaced, and diuretics such as Mannitol and Frusemide are used to encourage a good renal output. Dehydration must be avoided and adequate intravenous fluids given in addition to blood transfusion which is replacing blood loss. It is usual in uncomplicated cases to load the patient with extra fluid by giving 1 litre of Hartmann's solution in 3 hours prior to the operation.

Operative Technique

The operation is performed through a vertical incision as long as possible, i.e., from the costal margin to the symphysis pubis. A large self-retaining retractor is inserted. Most surgeons pack off the small intestine to gain access to the aneurysm. An older technique is to bring all the intestines outside the abdomen. This usually results in severe post-operative paralytic ileus even if the intestines are protected in a polythene bag.

The aorta must be isolated and clamped above the aneurysm. If the aneurysm is leaking this step must be accomplished as rapidly as possible. Clamps are also placed on the main arteries below the aneurysm. This usually means the two common iliac arteries. The surgeon always tries to do only that which is absolutely necessary to reconstruct the aorta and iliac arteries (Fig. 12.2). If the aneurysm extends to involve the iliac artery a bifurcation graft will be needed. Only one artery comes off the front of the aorta. This is the inferior mesenteric artery which has to be ligated. The blood supply to the colon is maintained via collateral arteries. In addition there are paired lumbar arteries which arise from the back of the aorta, but these cannot be reached and ligated at this stage of the operation.

Once the aorta has been clamped above, and the iliac arteries below the aneurysm it is possible to incise the aneurysm and to evacuate blood and clot which it contains. If there is back bleeding from the lumbar arteries they are sutured within the aneurysm. The woven dacron graft which has been pre-clotted is now sutured into the defect. The surgeon usually does this with 20 or 25 mm needles which are easier to manage than the smaller needles used on peripheral arteries.

Post-operative observations and Management

An operation for ruptured aortic aneurysm usually has a more complicated post-operative course than an elective operation, and such cases are usually managed in the intensive care unit.

1. Peripheral Circulation

It is necessary to observe the circulation in the feet and legs. Thrombus may form in the leg arteries during the time that the main arteries are clamped and the circulation arrested. Following surgery the feet should become warm and pink. The foot pulses are often palpable. Pallor of the feet may be due to vasospasm. Any deterioration in the circulation shown by coolness, blue discoloration, or loss of foot pulses should be reported. Pulse volume recordings are the only satisfactory way of assessing the circulation.

2. Blood and Fluid Transfusion

When large-volume transfusions of blood are involved it is easy to over-load the circulation with too much blood, and also to under-transfuse.

Fifteen-minute interval readings of the pulse rate and blood pressure are essential. Generally a rapid pulse and low blood pressure is an indication for further transfusion of blood.

3. Central Venous Pressure

A more accurate technique for assessment of the need for more or less blood transfusion is measurement of the central venous pressure.

The central venous pressure is measured by placing a plastic catheter in the superior vena cava. The catheter may be inserted through a vein in the arm or into the subclavian vein in the neck. The central venous pressure line is connected to a bottle of isotonic intravenous fluid and a three-way tap which is connected to a tube for measurement of pressure (Fig. 13.1). The intravenous fluid is

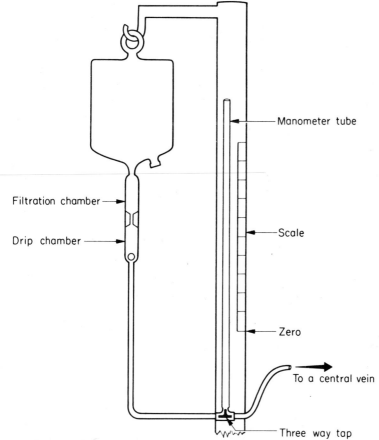

Fig. 13.1 This illustrates the technique used for measuring central venous pressure. The infusion bag is connected with a three-way tap. The manometer tube is taped to the drip stand and a centimetre scale is stuck onto the drip stand alongside the tube. The infusion stand is moved up or down until zero on the scale is level with the mid-axilla of the patient.

kept running at a slow rate to keep the line open. Some surgeons recommend taking the sternum as zero but the mid-axillary line is more commonly used and is more accurate. To get the point a spirit level is used from the mid-axillary line and the manometer tube is placed with zero on the scale at this level.

To measure the pressure the three-way tap is turned so that the manometer tube is filled from the intravenous set. The tap is then turned again so that fluid runs from the manometer tube to the patient. The level in the manometer tube will stop falling when equal to the central venous pressure. When zero is taken as the mid-axillary line the pressure should be within the range 3–10 cm of water.

There is always a risk of infection in an intravenous catheter left in for a period of time. The manometer and intravenous set should be changed daily and this route should not be used for injections which may introduce infection.

4. Urine Output

The state of hydration and renal function may be assessed by renal output. A catheter is placed in the bladder and the output measured hourly. The aim is to have a urinary output of 1·5–2 ml per minute.

5. Abdominal Complications

As the operation on the aorta is done transperitoneally some ileus is inevitable. During the period of non-function the intestines tend to dilate and fill with intestinal fluid. The patient will need intravenous therapy to combat the fluid loss, and a Ryle's tube to prevent vomiting of the stomach contents. The Ryle's tube is put on continuous drainage and the volume of gastric output is measured and charted.

When the intestinal function recovers the patient will pass flatus, and intestinal sounds may be heard with the stethoscope. At this point the intravenous infusion and gastric suction are stopped and the patient put onto oral fluids.

14
Dissecting Aneurysm

The lesion which causes dissection is a split in the aorta near its origin from the heart. The split is in the interior of the aorta but only reaches part way through the middle part of the wall of the aorta (the media) (Fig. 14.1). Obviously, if the split were through the whole thickness

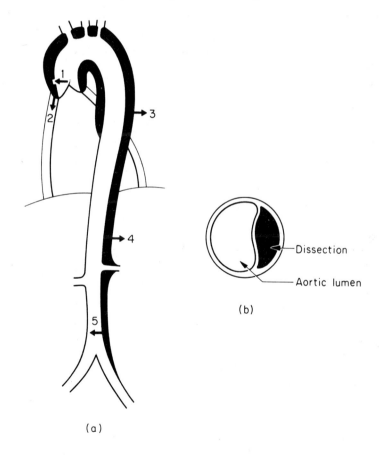

(b)

— Dissection

— Aortic lumen

(a)

Fig. 14.1 Dissecting aneurysm. (a) Distribution of dissection. (b) Transverse section of aorta. Arrows indicate: 1, rupture giving rise to dissection; 2, rupture of dissection into pericardium; 3, rupture into pleural cavity; 4, rupture into abdominal cavity; 5, rupture back into lumen of aorta—spontaneous recovery.

of the aorta the patient would immediately bleed to death. As the split is into the media the blood escapes from the lumen of the aorta into its wall where, under aortic pressure, it gradually dissects a tunnel to carry the blood within the aortic wall giving rise to a 'twin-bore' aorta as illustrated in Fig. 14.1. As the new channel of blood passes branches of the aorta these may be compressed. Compression of the carotid may cause cerebral symptoms, and of the subclavian artery may cause symptoms of ischaemia in the hand. As the dissection proceeds down the main thoracic aorta the patient usually complains of severe back pain. Compression of one or both renal arteries may give rise to signs of renal failure, and compression of an iliac artery may cause symptoms of ischaemia in the leg.

Many cases occur in elderly patients with atherosclerosis, and in these it is likely that atheromatous degeneration is the cause of the disease. However, the disease may also occur in younger patients who have an abnormality of the media predisposing to rupture. One such condition is a hereditary disease known as Marfan's syndrome which may be complicated by dissecting or fusiform aneurysm of the aorta at a young age.

Most patients have high blood pressure which may be a contributory cause.

Course and Prognosis

Dissection of the aorta is a particularly fatal disease. Death is usually from haemorrhage resulting from rupture of the dissecting blood through the outer coat of the aorta. As the first part of the aorta is within the pericardial sac it is possible for the dissection to rupture into the pericardium. The pericardium is a fibrous bag which encases the heart. When the dissection ruptures into the pericardium and fills the sac with blood the heart is compressed. The important result is that the heart is unable to receive blood from the great veins because the receiving chambers (atria) cannot expand. This effectively arrests the circulation and causes death. Compression of the heart by blood in the pericardium is called tamponade.

Death from haemorrhage may result from rupture of the dissection into the chest or abdominal cavities, and death is usual within the first 48 hours.

Very rarely the dissection may rupture back into the aorta. This at once takes the pressure out of the dissection which stops progressing. Such an event may be followed by full recovery. The patient is left with a twin-bore aorta.

Clinical Features

The outstanding clinical feature is the sudden onset of very severe pain in the chest and back. Many cases are incorrectly diagnosed as having a coronary thrombosis as the clinical picture is initially similar. The characteristic feature of dissection is that as the dissection proceeds a variety of new symptoms and signs appear consistent with narrowing or occlusion of branches of the aorta. Patients may be admitted to hospital with acute ischaemia of the upper or lower limb or with hemiplegia.

Diagnosis

The surgeon usually diagnoses this condition on clinical grounds. Plain radiography usually shows widening of the thoracic aorta. Aortography is probably unwise and is not generally done.

Conservative Treatment

The high mortality following attempts at surgical treatment of aortic dissection has led to its replacement by medical measures in many centres, though the mortality remains very high.

The main aspect of medical treatment is to reduce the blood pressure in an attempt to control further dissection and prevent rupture into the pericardium. A fatal outcome is usual but the patient is saved from a useless and major operation.

Surgical Treatment

The observation that some cases underwent spontaneous cure as a result of rupture of the dissection back into the aortic lumen led surgeons to try to imitate this. The mortality of this operation is very high and does not always prevent later external rupture of the dissection and death.

An alternative is to resect a part of the thoracic or abdominal aorta and to replace it with a dacron graft. At this operation the upper anastomosis is made to the outer layer of the aorta so that the lumen of the aorta and of the dissection open into the graft. When the surgeon turns to the lower end he begins by running a continuous suture round the aorta to close the dissected layer. The dacron graft is then sutured to the repaired aorta below.

When this operation is performed on the lower abdominal aorta compression of the renal arteries may not be relieved. However, if the operation is performed on the thoracic aorta there are additional and serious hazards. If the thoracic aorta is clamped for more than 20 minutes there will be irreversible damage to the kidneys and spinal cord. If it is decided that the dacron graft is to be put into the thoracic aorta some form of tube bypass must be arranged so that the kidneys, spinal cord, and other structures receive a blood supply during the period of clamping of the aorta. At the completion of the graft operation the bypass is removed. This is a very major undertaking.

15
Cerebrovascular Disease

Anatomy (Fig. 15.1)

The brain receives its blood supply through four arteries which pass through the neck to the brain.

Carotid Arteries

The origin of the two common carotid arteries differs on the two sides. The left common carotid takes origin directly from the aorta between the innominate and the left subclavian arteries. The right common carotid arises from the innominate artery. The innominate artery is the first major branch of the aorta and divides into the right subclavian and the right common carotid artery. The two common carotid arteries run up through the neck and divide at about the upper border of the larynx into the internal and external carotid arteries. The external carotid artery remains outside the skull and its branches are distributed to the thyroid gland, face, jaws, and scalp. The internal carotid has no branches outside the skull. After entering the skull it takes part in the anastomotic circle between the two internal carotid arteries and the two branches of the basilar artery which is called the circle of Willis and which lies between the base of the skull and the under surface of the brain.

Vertebral Arteries

The vertebral arteries are both branches of the subclavian artery. After a short course each vertebral artery enters the foramen in the transverse process of the sixth cervical vertebra. Each cervical vertebra has a foramen in its transverse process, and the vertebral artery ascends through these foramina and the intervening tissue and finally enters the skull through the foramen magnum. The two vertebral arteries then join to form the basilar artery which gives important branches to the base of the brain which contains nerve centres controlling the vital functions of life. The basilar artery then divides to form the two posterior cerebral arteries which join the back of the circle of Willis (Fig. 15.1).

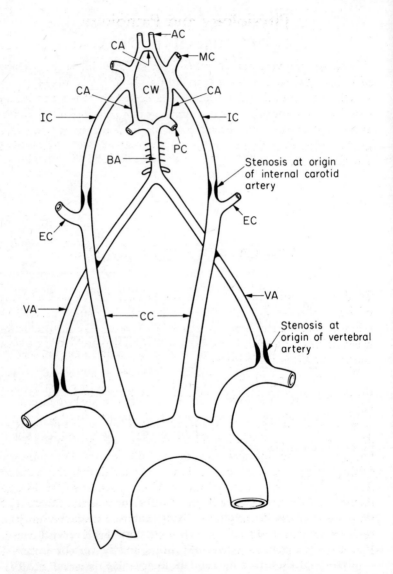

Fig. 15.1 Cerebral circulation showing common sites of atherosclerosis. Emboli from the carotid pass to the same side of the brain. Emboli from the vertebral arteries pass through the basilar artery and may reach either side of the brain. IC, internal carotid artery; EC, external carotid artery; CC, common carotid artery; VA, vertebral artery; BA, basilar artery; AC, anterior cerebral artery; MC, middle cerebral artery; PC, posterior cerebral artery; CA, communicating arteries; CW, circle of Willis.

Physiology and Pathology

The carotid and vertebral arteries supply the brain through the circle of Willis in which the blood from all four branches is mixed. If one vertebral or carotid artery becomes narrowed there is a possibility that flow from the other three arteries can compensate for this and so avoid ischaemia to the brain, particularly if the narrowing is a gradual process giving time for the increase in flow in the other arteries to take place.

Aneurysm of Circle of Willis

Small aneurysms sometimes form on the circle of Willis. The cause of these aneurysms is unknown but they are not caused by athero-sclerosis. These aneurysms sometimes rupture causing subarachnoid haemorrhage or serious brain damage if the aneurysm ruptures into and damages the brain itself.

Treatment of aneurysm of the circle of Willis is usually directed to the aneurysm, which is exposed and its neck occluded with a metal clip.

When the aneurysm is so placed that it is inaccessible or too dangerous to expose the carotid artery may be ligated in the neck. Ligation of the internal carotid usually lowers the pressure sufficiently to stop the bleeding but carries a risk that the reduced flow of blood may cause cerebral ischaemia. Lack of blood flow to the brain may cause a stroke if it is of sufficient severity. Ligation of the common carotid artery is less likely to cause a stroke because the cerebral circulation will continue through the internal carotid artery. Blood reaches the internal carotid through the generous collateral communication between the two external carotid arteries (Fig. 15.2). Prediction of the possibility of a stroke after ligation of the internal carotid artery is difficult but the operation becomes more dangerous in patients over 50 years.

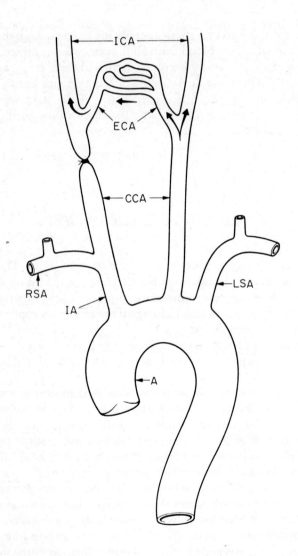

Fig. 15.2 Effect of ligation of common carotid artery. Circulation in internal carotid through anastomoses between right and left external carotid arteries (diagrammatic). ICA, internal carotid artery; ECA, external carotid artery; CCA, common carotid artery; RSA, right subclavian artery; LSA, left subclavian artery, IA, innominate artery; A, arch of aorta.

Atherosclerosis

Atherosclerotic plaques usually occur at bifurcations and particularly at the origin of the vertebral arteries and in the first 2 cm of the internal carotid artery (Fig. 15.1). Slight narrowing of one artery is unlikely to cause symptoms because of the collateral circulation at the circle of Willis. When the flow in the internal carotid artery is considerably reduced by atheromatous plaque the whole of the internal carotid artery may thrombose from its origin in the neck to its termination in the circle of Willis. This may so reduce the blood flow in the circle of Willis that the brain on that side becomes sufficiently ischaemic to cause a stroke.

A thrombus often forms on an atheromatous plaque and tiny fragments may break off from time to time. The common site for this is the first 2 cm of the internal carotid artery, and tiny fragments of thrombus are carried in the circulation to reach the brain where they finally lodge in a small artery in the brain substance causing a minor stroke.

Clinical Syndromes

1. Vertebrobasilar Ischaemia

Although the blood supply to the brain is through the circle of Willis the vertebral arteries mainly supply the back and base of the brain through the posterior cerebral arteries and the branches of the basilar artery (Fig. 15.1).

Reduction of blood flow in a vertebral artery or platelet thrombus emboli into the brain cause a variety of symptoms. There may be weakness and numbness in any of the limbs, blindness, double vision (diplopia), and giddiness (vertigo). The lack of localization to one side is because the two vertebral arteries join to form the centrally placed basilar artery. An embolus passing through this artery may pass to either side of the brain at the division of the basilar artery. The symptoms are usually transitory and pass off in a few hours.

2. Carotid Ischaemia

The carotid artery mainly supplies the cerebral hemispheres of the brain. Symptoms of ischaemia are usually on one side of the brain, causing weakness or numbness on the opposite side of the body. Difficulty in speaking (dysphasia) is present if the side of the brain responsible for speech is affected. In right-handed people this is generally the left side of the brain. There may be complete loss of vision in one eye as a result of an embolus passing through the main artery to the eye (ophthalmic artery).

Transient Attacks

The characteristic feature of these attacks is that there is sudden onset of symptoms and signs of a minor stroke which pass within an hour. The attacks tend to be recurrent and, in these circumstances, the diagnosis of carotid or vertebral artery stenosis should be considered. If the attacks are allowed to continue the function of the brain gradually deteriorates and recovery between attacks becomes less complete. Sometimes a complete stroke results from repeated transient attacks. This may be due to recurrent emboli into the brain or to a complete occlusion of the internal carotid artery.

Cerebral Haemorrhage

Not all strokes are due to carotid or vertebral artery atherosclerosis. In some patients a stroke is due to cerebral haemorrhage but this is usually quite a different presentation with paralysis and loss of consciousness. The stroke is due to brain damage caused by a haemorrhage arising from a ruptured artery in the brain substance.

Investigation of Transient Ischaemic Attacks

Remember that atherosclerosis is a generalized disease which may present in a variety of special ways. The patient has a full clinical examination with particular reference to the vascular system. There may be other signs of atherosclerosis such as arterial occlusions in the leg or an aortic aneurysm, and there may be a history of angina or coronary thrombosis caused by atherosclerosis in the coronary arteries. It is usual to evaluate this further by doing an ECG. In the neck the surgeon may be able to hear a bruit (murmur) caused by blood rushing through the stenosis of the internal carotid artery.

Arteriography

The special test which is done to diagnose the condition precisely and anatomically is arteriography. This is described in Chapter 3.

There are a variety of techniques and surgeons vary in their choice. The surgeon may ask for a carotid arteriogram on the side affected, or sometimes for a bilateral carotid arteriogram. When full information concerning the carotid and vertebral arteries is required the surgeon will order an aortic arch aortogram which will show all four arteries. However, this is a much more serious undertaking and is not requested as a matter of routine.

Medical Treatment

Drugs which Oppose Platelet Function

There are certain drugs which have some effect in preventing the aggregation of platelets. Aspirin and Dipyridamole have been used but the results are uncertain. The object is to prevent the formation of the platelet thrombus which is responsible for the emboli.

Anticoagulation Therapy

Many neurologists employ long term anticoagulation therapy after the first ischaemic attack. It is hoped that propagation and recurrent thrombi will be prevented. There is evidence that the incidence of recurrent minor strokes is substantially reduced by long-term anticoagulent therapy but there is a small incidence of haemorrhage. It is usual to begin treatment with Heparin and to change this to Coumarin for long-term out-patient treatment.

Surgical Treatment

This is indicated when the patient is reasonably fit and is shown by carotid arteriography to have a localized lesion which is suitable for surgical treatment. The common lesion at the origin of the internal carotid artery is that generally suitable for surgical treatment.

Principle of Surgical Treatment

The main problem concerns the temporary interruption of blood flow through one carotid artery while the atheromatous plaque is removed. It is known that the higher centres of the brain cannot tolerate deprivation of oxygen for more than 3 minutes. Cardiac arrest for more than 3 minutes will be followed by permanent brain damage. It is possible that clamping the internal carotid for more than 3 minutes might have a similar effect on that side of the brain, and for many years the operation was performed under

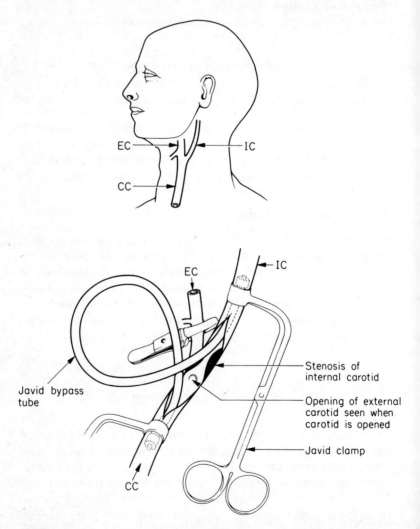

Fig. 15.3 Use of bypass in surgical treatment of carotid stenosis. The artery has been opened and the bypass is in place. CC, common carotid; EC, external carotid; IC, internal carotid.

hypothermia. In this technique the body temperature is lowered to 30 °C. This may be done by immersion of the anaesthetized patient into a cold water bath. At lower body temperature the brain can withstand ischaemia for longer periods but the exact time is uncertain.

The modern technique is to insert a plastic bypass between the common carotid artery and the internal carotid artery so that a normal circulation is maintained during the operation (Fig. 15.3).

Operation for Carotid Stenosis

After induction of anaesthesia the patient is placed on the operating table with the head turned away from the side of the operation. A long incision is made in the neck. It runs from behind the angle of the jaw down the front of the sternomastoid muscle to just above the sternum. The surgeon dissects out the three carotid arteries. The patient is now fully heparinized by the anaesthetist so that clotting of blood does not take place when the clamps are in position, nor in the plastic bypass tube. Atraumatic artery clamps are then put onto the three arteries. The clamp on the external carotid artery remains throughout the operation. With the clamps in position it is possible to make an incision in the internal carotid artery about 3 cm in length. A special bypass plastic tube is then inserted (Fig. 15.3) and the original clamps on the common carotid and internal carotid arteries are removed to allow blood to flow again. The plastic tube has a flange at each end and is held in place with special clamps (Javid). The surgeon may then proceed to remove the atheromatous plaque without any restriction on time. When the plaque and thrombus is satisfactorily removed a vein patch is placed on the incision in the carotid artery to prevent narrowing, and the bypass tube is removed. The wound is closed with a suction drain.

Post-operative Observations

Local Observations

Although this operation is usually free from complications the usual local observations for haematoma or external bleeding are made as with any vascular operation. Haematoma in the neck should be reported at once as there is always a risk that it may cause compression of the trachea. The wound should be inspected at 15-minute intervals when the pulse and blood pressure are also taken.

Cerebral Observations

With good technique there should be no interference with cerebral function. When the brain has suffered ischaemia or embolism its function may be impaired. Following the operation the patient should gradually regain consciousness. Failure to regain consciousness may be an indication of brain damage. The pupils should also be observed. They should be small and react to light. Large pupils not reacting to light are an indication of serious brain damage.

The nurse may also observe paralysis on one side of the body.

Vertebral Stenosis

Surgical treatment of vertebral stenosis is sometimes undertaken. The origin of the vertebral artery is very inaccessible and also narrow so that most surgeons are reluctant to undertake this operation.

The Subclavian Steal Syndrome

The term 'steal' is used in artery surgery when as a result of an occlusion or perhaps a large diameter graft, blood passes in a direction which it finds easier, so stealing blood flow from going in the normal direction. A good but rare example of this is the subclavian steal. In this condition there is an occlusion of the first part of the left subclavian artery. The subclavian artery then receives its blood from the left vertebral artery where the direction of flow is reversed (Fig. 15.4). In effect, the subclavian artery is stealing blood which would normally ascend in the vertebral artery to the brain.

Occlusion of the first part of the subclavian artery may produce three sets of symptoms:

1. The symptoms and signs of ischaemia including gangrene in the hand or fingers.
2. Signs of cerebral ischaemia such as dizzy attacks and vertigo.
3. A combination of brain and arm symptoms.

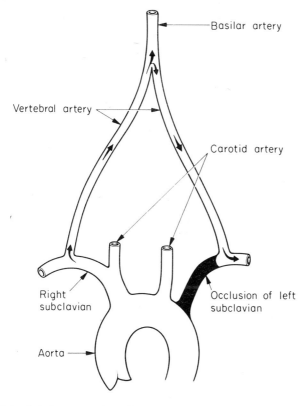

Fig. 15.4 Subclavian steal syndrome. The left subclavian is occluded and steals blood from the left vertebral artery, which has a reversed flow

The treatment of the subclavian steal syndrome is surgical. The first part of the subclavian artery is in the chest and can be reached by a postero-lateral thoracotomy. The exact technique for treatment depends on the exact situation but it is usually possible to bypass the occlusion with a short dacron graft.

16
Diabetic Gangrene

Diabetes mellitus remains a serious disease, and vascular complications are frequently seen. Some diabetic patients have high
levels of blood cholesterol, and atherosclerosis is often severe and
diffuse. However, the relationship of diabetes and vascular disease is
variable. Three distinct clinical presentations must be recognized:

1. Senile atherosclerosis with gangrene. The patient also has
   diabetes, usually mild, but the diabetes is coincidental and
   bears no relationship to the gangrene which is managed as an
   uncomplicated case of atheromatous gangrene.
2. Typical diabetic gangrene of the foot with marked ischaemic
   changes. In this case the gangrenous and infected foot is
   primarily due to diabetes but the arterial occlusions and
   ischaemia contribute to the problem and need to be taken
   into account in the management.
3. Uncomplicated diabetic gangrene of the foot may occur in a
   youngish person with normal foot pulses and no ischaemic
   changes. Certain features of diabetic gangrene make it very
   characteristic so that the diagnosis is often apparent to the
   surgeon on simple clinical observations.

Diabetic Neuropathy

The peripheral nerves are often affected in diabetics. The usual
nerves to be affected are those to the foot, and the first changes to be
noticed are loss of vibration sense and of the ankle jerk. Later the
sensory loss extends to include loss of all sensation on the foot. This
loss of sensation is highly important to the diabetic as the foot may
be injured in a variety of ways without the patient being aware of
the fact, and such an injury acts as a portal of entry for bacteria. It is
well known that infection in any part of the body is inclined to
spread more rapidly in a diabetic and this is also true of infection of
the foot.

The foot may be injured by such a simple accident as stepping on a sharp object. Also the foot may be damaged in course of chiropody involving treatment of nails and corns. In the normal subject pain prevents injury but in the diabetic with neuropathy the condition may resemble those existing after injection of a local anaesthetic. Finally the diabetic is particularly prone to pressure ulceration. The anaesthetic foot is not moved because it is not uncomfortable, and when lying in bed a pressure sore 4 cm in diameter may form on the outer aspect of the heel.

There is one favourable aspect of the neurotrophic complication of diabetes. This is that the patient with dry senile gangrene does not have the relentless rest pain which is usually so characteristic of the condition, and amputation is not forced on the patient because of pain.

Infection

Diabetics are particularly prone to infection. When infection enters the foot there are three characteristic features:

1. It tends to spread rapidly through the foot, running along the fascial planes and tendon sheaths.
2. There is a tendency for bones, especially the phalanges and metatarsals, to become involved with infection. The surgeon will take X-rays to locate bone infection. Pieces of bone frequently die as a result of infection, and after some weeks these fragments become separated from the adjacent living bone. A fragment of dead bone is called a sequestrum and an infection will not heal up until all sequestra are discharged or removed.
3. Infection with gas-forming organisms is quite common. Gas bubbles may be seen coming from the wound or may be felt in the foot by light palpation. This sensation is given the descriptive clinical term of crepitus. Bubbles of gas in the tissues may also be seen on radiographs which have the advantage of showing gas deep in the tissues where it cannot be felt. Gas infection of the subcutaneous tissues is not usually serious but when infection with *Clostridium welchii* (a bacterium which produces gas) involves the muscle bellies in the foot and calf the patient may die with septicaemia.

Clinical Management

1. Care of Feet in Diabetes

Any diabetic patient may suffer the complication of severe infection in the foot. Preventative measures are directed to regular washing of the feet followed by careful drying and the use of an antiseptic powder. Great care should be taken concerning the formation of pressure ulcers particularly after the patient is fitted with new shoes. The patient must also be warned of the dangers of careless cutting of the nails or of corns. If necessary he should be referred to a good chiropodist for regular care of the feet.

2. Management of Diabetic Gangrene

In the typical diabetic gangrene the foot becomes acutely inflamed with redness spreading over a wide area. It is important to try and get some localization of this infection by general measures and the patient is treated with bed rest and broad spectrum antibiotics. During this period the diabetes will go out of control and an increase in the dose of insulin will be required.

Incisions to drain pus will eventually be needed. At this operation sloughs consisting of dead fascia and tendons may be removed along with bone sequestra. The wound is left open to drain and will need daily irrigation and dressing with an antiseptic such as Eusol. The dressings are often painless because of the neuropathy. These cases are often slow in healing. Both the surgeon and patient need to be patient as too early surgery may spread the infection and eventually lead to loss of even more tissue.

3. Amputation

In cases in which *Clostridium welchii* is cultured from the wound and in which the muscles are involved with the infection the patient may become desperately ill. Infection spreads rapidly and the patient will die from septic shock unless an early decision is made to amputate the leg above the infection.

4. Vein or Dacron Graft Operations

In diabetic cases there is a tendency for the arterial disease to be severe below the level of the knee so that grafting is impossible.

Grafts are indicated in a few cases where there is occlusion of the femoral artery combined with diabetic gangrene of the foot. The operation should not be performed until the acute stage of the infection has been overcome.

Prognosis

Patients are likely to get recurrent attacks of diabetic gangrene and infection in the foot resulting in gradual loss of toes and foot in repeated attacks. Also the disease will occur in the other foot. With care and conservative treatment the feet can be conserved over many years, but hasty and ill-judged surgery can lead to early amputation which may later be repeated on the second side.

17
Buerger's Disease

Buerger's disease is of unknown aetiology, although it is made much worse by cigarette smoking, and if a patient with Buerger's disease can be persuaded to stop smoking the disease will be largely controlled if not actually arrested. It was described in 1908 by Buerger who called it thromboangiitis obliterans because of the formation of obliterating thrombus in the arteries and veins accompanied by inflammatory changes in the vessel wall.

Buerger's disease characteristically occurs in young men. It is virtually unknown in women. It may affect the arteries of the upper limb and the viscera as well as those in the legs, but the distal arteries in the legs are always affected first. In the legs the smaller, distal arteries are affected in contrast to atherosclerosis where the larger proximal arteries are usually affected first. Attacks of superficial thrombophlebitis often precede arterial thrombosis.

The disease is rare and difficult to define with precision. There is usually some excess of sympathetic tone. The sympathetic nerves control the peripheral blood flow and also secretion of sweat glands so that these patients show the two effects of increased sympathetic tone. The hands and feet are pale and subject to sudden increases in pallor which is called Raynaud's phenomenon. The effect on the sweat glands is demonstrated by excessive perspiration. This is particularly marked in the feet where the moist soggy skin easily gets infected with fungi. The characteristic appearance of the feet is that they are pale, sweating, and affected by interdigital fungal infection.

Race

At one time it was thought that the disease occurred mainly in Jews. It is likely that this is because Buerger worked in a Jewish Hospital in New York where most of his patients were Jewish. At the present time it seems that there may be a slight preponderance of Jews but there is no marked racial bias.

Clinical Presentation

The patient is a male, under 40 years of age, with cool, sweating feet and hands, and often suffering from interdigital fungal infection in the feet.

Venous Involvement

There may be a history of phlebitis or it may be a feature at the time of presentation. A superficial vein anywhere may be affected. Commonly the patient complains of a painful lump in the leg, and examination shows this to be a vein which is the subject of thrombophlebitis. The vein is solid and tender to palpation. It also shows the changes of inflammation—heat, redness and swelling.

Arterial Involvement

This nearly always begins in the peripheral arteries so that the arterial effects are peripheral in contrast to the proximal disease and effects seen in atherosclerosis.

Intermittent Claudication

When the arteries of the foot (plantar arteries) are thrombosed the flow to the muscles of the sole of the foot is diminished and the patients complain of pain in the sole of the foot on walking. Characteristically this pain is relieved by rest. This is called intermittent claudication, and plantar claudication is a characteristic feature of Buerger's disease.

Gangrene

When the digital arteries are affected the toe may be completely ischaemic and develop gangrene. The characteristic feature of gangrene of the toes in Buerger's disease is that the foot has a good blood supply and the foot pulses are present. Again this is in contrast with atherosclerosis in which gangrene of the toe is caused by proximal arterial disease and the foot pulses are absent. Gangrene is always a very distressing and painful event, usually preventing sleep.

Investigations

The diagnosis is generally a clinical one and special investigations such as arteriography are unnecessary. If such an X-ray is done it only confirms the process of distal arterial obstruction.

Treatment

Smoking

It is absolutely essential that the patient should completely give up smoking. There is no doubt that many patients with Buerger's disease have a strong addiction to cigarette smoking and it may be advisable to admit them to hospital and to use tranquillizing drugs.

Sympathectomy

Lumbar or upper dorsal sympathectomy is particularly useful in cases of Buerger's disease which have not yet progressed to gangrene. The foot will become warm and dry and rest pain may be relieved. It is wise to try to avoid bilateral lumbar sympathectomy in those patients who are young men as it may cause impotence.

Amputations

Because the arterial disease is distal it is possible to amputate a gangrenous toe with good expectation of primary healing. The surgeon always makes two equal flaps as the end of a single long flap is likely to die. It is usual to try and assist the blood supply to the flaps and to help healing by doing a lumbar sympathectomy at the same time as the amputation. When a toe is amputated some surgeons try to avoid sutures and bring the skin edges together with 'Steristrips' which are non-traumatic.

Prognosis

There is no doubt that the disease can be controlled by sympathectomy and minor amputation, and that further progress can be arrested provided the patient can give up cigarette smoking. If the patient continues to smoke the disease will progress proximally in spite of sympathectomy, and more proximal amputation of both upper and lower limb will be required.

Follow-up studies show that there is little effect on the expectation of life, which differs little from normal expectancy.

18
Raynaud's Disease, Raynaud's Phenomenon, and Allied Diseases

Maurice Raynaud described what is now known as Raynaud's disease in 1862. A variety of clinical conditions may give rise to symptoms somewhat similar to those of primary Raynaud's disease and the term Raynaud's phenomenon has been applied to these.

Raynaud's Disease

This is a disease which primarily affects the hands of young women although the feet may also be affected. It also occurs in pre-menopausal women in a modified form. The appearance of the disease at these two ages, and almost entirely in women, has given rise to the suggestion that sex hormones play some part in its causation.

The basic clinical feature of Raynaud's disease is the sudden constriction of tiny blood vessels (arterioles) leading to the skin of the fingers. In nearly all cases the sudden constriction is triggered by exposure to cold, but in about 25% of cases intense emotion has a similar effect. Both hands are usually equally affected. The incidents which are typical of Raynaud's disease occur in three phases.

1. With sudden acute spasm in the small vessels and arrest of the arterial circulation the fingers become white in colour.
2. After some minutes the spasm begins to pass off, letting some blood through to the fingers. As they have been starved of blood and oxygen the first blood to pass through to the fingers quickly gives up its oxygen and becomes blue in colour. The second stage is that the fingers become blue in colour.
3. The spasm disappears completely. Because of the deprivation of blood flow for some minutes the finger undergoes reactive hyperaemia. This is a normal response to temporary ischaemia and is typically seen when a tourniquet is removed. During the period of circulatory arrest the part

continues to live and metabolize, and the products of metabolism which are normally carried away in the blood remain locally in the tissues. Here they cause dilatation of all the blood vessels so that when the spasm is relaxed and blood re-enters the part it becomes red, swollen and painful as the blood fills all the enlarged, dilated blood vessels.

Raynaud's disease is very common in young women and shows a tendency to gradually become less severe. Most cases remain of nuisance value and are not a serious disability. In a very small proportion of cases the repeated attacks of vasoconstriction and ischaemia cause permanent effects. The skin and pulp of the finger begin to atrophy. As the disease progresses the small arteries (arterioles) may, in a small percentage of cases, become occluded and gangrene of the finger tip results.

Raynaud's Phenomenon

Raynaud's phenomenon may be the first sign of some underlying vascular disorder, and it is often said that one cannot diagnose Raynaud's disease with certainty until it has been present without signs of underlying vascular disease for at least 2 years.

In secondary Raynaud's phenomenon the presenting features of sensitivity to cold shown by initial blanching of the fingers, followed by blueness, and then reactive hyperaemia is similar to that of primary Raynaud's disease. In primary Raynaud's disease the underlying cause remains obscure. In secondary Raynaud's phenomenon certain underlying diseases play a part, as yet unknown, in the presentation. The common diseases which cause Raynaud's phenomenon are:

1. Buerger's disease (Thromboangiitis obliterans). When a young man presents with the Raynaud's phenomenon, primary Raynaud's disease is unlikely. In this age and sex it is likely that signs of Buerger's disease will appear within two years.

2. Atherosclerosis. When the syndrome occurs in older men or women it may be the precursor of generalized atherosclerosis.

3. Anatomical abnormalities in the neck such as cervical rib may cause Raynaud's phenomenon.

Treatment of Raynaud's Disease

In its milder form the management of Raynaud's disease consists of commonsense measures to avoid exposure to cold. Thick gloves and, if necessary, fur-lined boots should be worn in cold weather. Immersion of the hands in cold water is to be avoided. No drug treatment has up to now proved of any value at all.

Surgical Treatment

In very severe cases causing disability or threatening gangrene of the finger tip, great benefit can be obtained from the operation of upper dorsal sympathectomy which can be performed on both sides at the same operation. As the patients are young the axillary approach, described in Chapter 5, is preferred as, in addition to giving good, safe access to the sympathetic chain, the scar is in a cosmetically acceptable position. Although the initial result is dramatic, the effects of sympathectomy become less marked in a few months. However some permanent benefit is always obtained.

The management of Raynaud's phenomenon is identical with that of primary Raynaud's disease. However, it is not usually so severe and sympathectomy is not often required.

Scleroderma

As a result of recurrent attacks of Raynaud's phenomenon the skin of the fingers may become thick and hardened—the condition known as scleroderma. There is another condition of generalized scleroderma involving similar changes in the skin of the mouth and oesophagus, but it is unlikely that scleroderma affecting the fingers in a case of Raynaud's disease will ever become generalized.

Acrocyanosis

The literal translation of acrocyanosis is blue ends. The affliction occurs particularly in young women often with fat legs. The most likely explanation of the condition is that there is poor blood flow in the skin of the hands and feet which are permanently blue and cold. The hands are usually affected first, but in many cases the feet and legs are also blue and cold. The condition in no way resembles Raynaud's disease as the episodic attacks of blanching, so typical of Raynaud's disease, do not occur.

Treatment is usually confined to general measures of keeping warm, and sympathectomy is rarely indicated.

Cervical Rib

Anatomy

There are normally twelve ribs attached posteriorly to the 12 dorsal vertebrae. The main nerves to the arm originate from the spinal cord in the neck and emerge behind a muscle called scalenus anterior, cross the top of the first rib, lie between the first rib and the clavicle, and enter the axilla. This nerve plexus is called the brachial plexus. The main artery and vein are connected to great vessels in the chest. The subclavian vein comes from the axilla, crosses the top of the first rib, passes in front of the scalenus muscle and then dips behind the inner end of the first rib to enter the chest carrying blood towards the

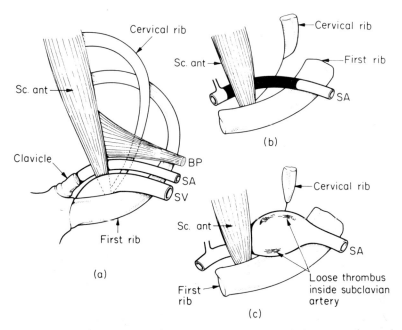

Fig. 18.1 (a) Cervical rib. BP, brachial plexus; SA, subclavian artery; SV, subclavian vein; Sc. Ant, scalenus anterior muscle. Vascular complications: (b) Thrombosis of subclavian artery. (c) Aneurysm of subclavian artery with thrombus.

heart. The subclavian artery leaves the chest, passes behind the scalenus anterior muscle, and accompanies the nerves to the arm across the top of the rib into the arm (Fig. 18.1).

When this anatomy is normal the main blood vessels and nerves are not likely to get damaged by compression or kinking.

Anatomy of Cervical Rib

A cervical rib is an additional rib which arises from the seventh or lowest cervical vertebra. It runs forward above the first rib and is usually attached to it at about the same point as the scalenus anterior muscle. Sometimes the rib is complete from end to end but much more often the rib consists of bone for a variable distance and the anterior part is made of fibrous tissue. Probably a cervical rib causes no trouble in 90% of cases in which it is present. The cervical rib and scalenus anterior muscle make a V-shaped gap through which the brachial plexus and subclavian artery must pass, and it is here that compression or kinking may occur.

Neurological Complications

These may comprise tingling in the distribution of the lowest part of the brachial plexus. This causes tingling along the inner side of the forearm and in the hand. The brachial plexus is certainly in the cleft between the cervical rib and the muscle but it is now thought that nerve symptoms are rarely caused by a cervical rib. Many people, especially in middle age, complain of tingling in the hand and it is now thought that this is usually due to arthritis of the cervical spine causing pressure on the nerve roots. If an X-ray shows a cervical rib to be present it is probably an incidental finding.

Vascular Complications

Although vascular complications are rare there is no doubt that they occasionally occur. The fact that compression of the subclavian artery may take place is illustrated by the observation that in certain positions of the arm the pulse disappears from the wrist. Repeated injury to the subclavian artery over a period of years may so damage it that the wall is weakened and the artery dilates to form an aneurysm. Small fragments of thrombus formed in the aneurysm may be thrown off to form minute emboli in the hand. Repeated attacks of acute ischaemia may eventually cause gangrene of a finger tip.

Another complication of repeated trauma is that the main subclavian artery may undergo thrombosis. Luckily there is a good natural collateral circulation but the patient usually complains that the hand is cold and attacks of Raynaud's phenomenon are common (Fig. 18.1).

Treatment of Cervical Rib

It is, of course, important to be sure that the symptoms are due to the cervical rib and not to arthritis in the cervical spine. Most cases coming to surgical treatment today have vascular complications and these are undoubtedly due to the rib.

It is possible to resect the offending rib by making an incision in the neck above the collar bone. In cases in which there is a serious vascular complication such as aneurysm or thrombosis this will not be sufficient.

The subclavian artery is very inaccessible to surgery and reconstruction is rarely indicated. Luckily the coolness and Raynaud's phenomenon, which result from thrombosis of the subclavian artery, respond well to upper dorsal sympathectomy which is usually the operation of choice.

When the subclavian artery is aneurysmal, and the source of emboli to the hand, it should be treated by ligature of the artery proximal to the aneurysm so causing thrombosis of the aneurysm and preventing further emboli. This operation should be followed by sympathectomy to encourage the formation of a collateral circulation.

19
Arterial Injuries: (1) General Description

Causes

1. In England today road traffic accidents are the most common cause of a major arterial injury. When there is such an injury it is often part of a complicated trauma with injury in the head, chest, or abdomen. Many artery injuries caused by road traffic accidents are complicated by fractures.
2. In more violent societies knife and gunshot wounds account for a varying proportion of artery accidents. These injuries are usually more localized.
3. Safety measures in factories are now well advanced but industrial accidents still account for a proportion of injuries to arteries when safety precautions are disregarded.
4. Some operative procedures may accidentally damage an artery. This is particularly true of orthopaedic operations which are performed under a tourniquet. In this situation when an artery is damaged it is not revealed by serious haemorrhage until the tourniquet is released. Prolonged pressure by a retractor can also damage an artery sufficiently to cause a thrombosis. Considering the number of operations performed the number of injuries is very small.

Types of Injury (Fig. 19.1)

1. Complete severance of an artery is most commonly caused by knife wounds.
2. Partial severance of an artery causes considerable bleeding. When an artery is divided completely the ends retract and close, but a partial injury continues to bleed because the artery is in continuity and cannot retract. Such bleeding is usually contained in the body by fascial planes and a large haematoma forms in the tissue alongside the artery. The haematoma clots peripherally but a central part remains in

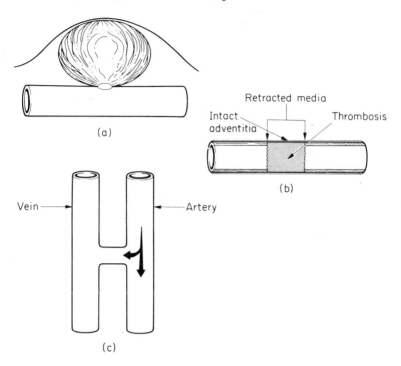

Fig. 19.1 Types of artery injury: (a) false aneurysm containing laminated thrombus; (b) medial tear; (c) arteriovenus fistula.

continuity with the arterial stream and the lump therefore pulsates. This lesion is called a pulsating haematoma or false aneurysm (page 62).

3. *Medial Tear.* The normal flow of blood in the blood vessels depends on the presence of an intact intima. When the intima is damaged clotting of the blood (thrombosis) is likely to take place. In the medial tear (Fig. 19.1) the artery receives a violent blow which transects the media and intima leaving the artery kept in continuity by the outer adventitial layer. The media is elastic and retracts leaving about 1–2 cm of artery which, although in continuity, does not have a lining of intima and soon thromboses. This condition gives all the usual signs of peripheral ischaemia, but when seen at operation the artery is intact. However, the medial tear is seen as a blue segment 1–2 cm in length and there is no pulse beyond this point. These artery injuries frequently complicate a major bone fracture.

4. *Arteriovenous Fistula.* A penetrating wound from a knife or bullet may pass between an artery and its accompanying vein, causing a partial injury to each. The arterial blood tends to flow into the low pressure vein at the site of injury, and the two vessels quickly heal leaving a communication or fistula. This fistula has interesting effects which depend on its size and the flow of blood.

(1) The blood flowing through the hole causes a vibration in the venous stream which is felt as a thrill over the vein and is heard as a murmur with the stethoscope.

(2) The arterial flow causes the vein to distend and to carry an increased volume of blood back to the right atrium. This extra blood has to be pumped by the heart and the heart output is increased. This may give rise to heart failure.

5. *Arterial Spasm.* This accompanies all types of artery injury and is part of the natural mechanism for the arrest of haemorrhage. When there is a serious injury to a limb, or more especially to the main artery in the limb, the smooth muscle which encircles the wall of the artery contracts to make the artery smaller in diameter. This is called a spasm. Obviously the flow of blood is reduced because the whole arterial system is reduced in size. Nature intends this mechanism to reduce the flow of blood in a severely injured part of the body and so naturally assist in the control of bleeding which is then more easily effected by platelets from the blood plugging small holes in the blood vessels and also by clotting of the blood where it is leaking from the damaged blood vessels.

An effect of spasm is to give rise to signs of reduced blood flow, and when spasm is severe it may cause sufficiently severe symptoms to be confused with those of an actual injury to the main artery. However, the effects of spasm are not usually quite as severe as those of an artery injury and they tend to pass off, while the effects of an injury persist or even get worse.

Clinical Appearance

The patient with an artery injury is usually in shock as a result of blood loss and associated injuries.

As far as the leg is concerned the changes depend on the type of injury.

HAEMATOMA. There is usually a large haematoma at the site of injury. The limb may be deformed because of a displaced fracture.

SIGNS OF ISCHAEMIA. These are usually present by the time the patient reaches hospital.

1. Skin Circulation. The reduction of blood flow in a limb will cause it to be pale in colour and within an hour the temperature of the skin is obviously below that of a normal leg. This is because there is a natural tendency for skin to cool because of insensible perspiration and radiation of heat. The temperature is normally kept up by the blood flow in the skin and when this is reduced the skin cools.

Later if the blood flow is considerably reduced the blood stagnating in the skin will have all its oxygen absorbed and the limb may have blotchy areas of blueness.

2. Lowered Blood Flow to Peripheral Nerves. The peripheral nerves transmit impulses. The motor nerves carry impulses from the brain which causes the activity of muscles in the leg and so movements of the limb. Messages from the skin pass through the sensory nerve fibres to the brain where they are interpreted as sensations of various kinds. Nerve fibres are very sensitive to a reduction in blood flow and the function of transmitting motor and sensory impulses is soon lost. This is seen in the patient in two ways.

When the sensory nerves fail to transmit impulses the skin becomes anaesthetic. The patient is asked to close his eyes and to say when he is touched on the limb.

The patient is also asked to move his toes and ankles. When the motor nerves are unable to function because of poor or absent blood supply the patient is unable to move his toe and other joints.

3. Peripheral Pulses. It is usual to try to palpate the peripheral pulses. In the leg this usually means the dorsalis pedis and posterior tibial pulses on the foot. However, this is not so important as the other signs. The foot pulses may be impalpable because of shock causing a low blood pressure or because of spasm of the arteries in the leg.

In addition, when there is a partial injury causing a pulsating haematoma, the peripheral pulses may still be present although the main artery has been damaged.

Associated Injuries

General

It is to be remembered that an arterial injury is often part of a major and complicated accident. In particular a road traffic accident may give rise to a head injury as well as abdominal and chest trauma. The same patient may have a fracture of the femur complicated by an artery injury.

When the patient comes into the accident department it is important that the priorities of management be properly observed. The first principle is to maintain life and there are two over-riding priorities:

1. To maintain the airway. In some types of chest injury respiration is inadequate, and intubation of the trachea to provide assisted respiration is the first priority. An anaesthetist may be the first person called on to save the patient's life.
2. Haemorrhage. Haemorrhage may be external or internal. In either event the loss of blood from the circulation causes shock. If there is insufficient blood in the blood vessels there is a generalized increase in output of sympathetic nerve impulses which cause contraction of the blood vessels. This makes the skin look pale. The sympathetic nerves also supply the sweat glands so that there is also an excess of perspiration in patients suffering from haemorrhage. In addition the pulse rate is rapid and the blood pressure reduced. Such a patient will die unless the blood volume is replaced and transfusion with plasma and blood must follow the establishment of an airway.

Only after the airway is established and replacement of blood loss commenced can the diagnosis of the injury be considered. General examination will include the central nervous system, chest, abdomen, and limbs where an artery injury may be suspected or diagnosed. Radiographs of the chest and any other area suspected of injury are taken.

Local

In the limbs the most important associated injury is a fracture. When a fracture occurs at a site close to a main artery the artery is at risk. The two common sites in the leg are a fracture of the lower third of the femur and of the upper end of the tibia. In the arm a fracture dislocation of the elbow joint or a fracture of the humerus just above the joint may damage the brachial artery.

The vein which accompanies a main artery is often severely damaged when the artery is injured. Veins are very difficult to repair, and it is fortunate that there are usually numerous alternative channels for venous return so that repair of damaged veins is not necessary.

The main nerves to the limb usually run near to the artery. Fortunately, they often escape injury but may be divided in penetrating injuries with glass or by stabbing. When the artery injury is associated with a fracture the nerves may be damaged as a result of stretching. These cases are unlikely to recover, but the divided nerve may be sutured with reasonable prospect of good recovery.

20
Arterial Injuries: (2) Management

A completely occluded main artery does not necessarily mean that the limb will be lost as the circulation can often be carried on through collateral vessels which develop. However, once the grave signs of anaesthesia and paralysis are present the limb is in peril and will be lost unless the circulation can be restored by an operation designed to repair the injured artery. In cases in which collateral circulation is adequate to preserve the limb it may still be advisable to repair the injured artery so that a normal limb is preserved. If the circulation is inadequate the limb is likely to function poorly, and in a child the leg with a subnormal circulation will not grow as fast as its normal fellow.

Of course, any injured artery which is bleeding internally to form a pulsating haematoma will need early surgical repair.

In general it is wise to operate and repair all injured arteries when this is technically possible, and as soon after the accident as circumstances permit. Although the operation should be performed as soon as possible no exact time can be given as the collateral circulation varies in different cases. However, once the patient shows anaesthesia and paralysis the artery must be repaired within 6 to 8 hours, as with this degree of ischaemia muscle necrosis is likely after the lapse of this period of time, and the leg will have to be amputated. An additional reason for early repair is that propagation thrombus will form in the artery below the occlusion after about 6 hours in the same way as it forms below an arterial embolus. In cases of embolus this can be prevented by the use of anticoagulants such as heparin, but anticoagulants are absolutely contra-indicated in traumatic cases because of the serious risk of haemorrhage from the injured part.

Principles of Operative Repair (Fig. 20.1)

1. Arteriogram

The diagnosis is usually made on clinical examination. However, the surgeon may wish to have exact details of the injury and in this case

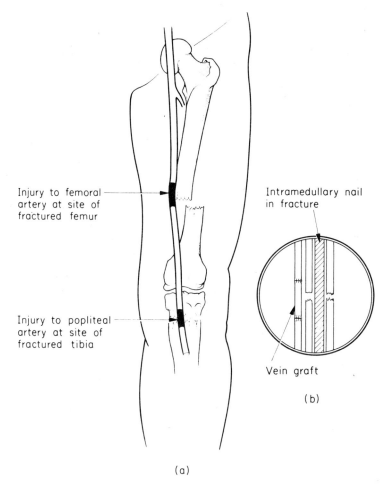

Injury to femoral artery at site of fractured femur

Intramedullary nail in fracture

Injury to popliteal artery at site of fractured tibia

Vein graft

(b)

(a)

Fig. 20.1 (a) Typical sites of medial tear injury complicating fracture. (b) Treatment by intramedullary nail and vein graft artery.

an arteriogram is done. This may considerably delay the operation, and to avoid too much delay the arteriogram is sometimes done on the operating table immediately before the operation.

2. Vein Patching or Grafting

When the artery is exposed it may be found that a vein graft is necessary to bridge an injured segment of artery. It is wise to remove a short length of saphenous vein from the opposite leg before exploring the injured artery. The vein is removed from the opposite leg as it is desirable not to interfere with venous drainage from the affected leg which may already have considerable venous damage. This piece of vein is distended with saline and preserved while the exposure of the injury is proceeding.

3. Immobilization of Fracture

In cases in which there is a complicating fracture, this must be soundly immobilized before the artery is repaired. The reason for this is that if the fracture is not immobilized movement may cause damage and bleeding or thrombosis at the site of an arterial repair. Fractures of the femur are often repaired by intramedullary nailing, and at other sites a steel plate may be used to fix the two pieces securely together.

4. Exposure and Repair of the Injured Artery

The exposure may be in whole or in part determined by an external wound. The artery is identified at the site of the injury and for 2 or 3 cm above and below that point. When all is exposed the artery is clamped with simple arterial clamps of the 'Bulldog' variety. Any associated vein injury is treated by ligature. In cases of medial tear and thrombosis the injured segment is excised and the defect bridged with a vein graft. When there is an incomplete lesion without thrombosis as might happen in a stabbing incident the artery is repaired with interrupted sutures. If it seems that the lumen of the artery will be narrowed a vein patch can be applied to widen it. Sutures of 5/0 prolene are ideal for repairs of this kind.

Arterial spasm may be a problem. It is difficult to overcome but unless relieved will reduce the flow of blood through a vein graft and may lead to early thrombosis of the graft. In addition the artery in spasm may be much smaller than the vein which is being inserted as a graft. Papaverine 2% is sometimes dabbed onto the artery in spasm but the effect is not usually dramatic. Another technique used by surgeons is to put a plastic catheter or cannula into the artery and to try and distend it with saline. Some surgeons attempt to widen the artery by inserting fine artery forceps and gently opening them.

If there is thrombus in the artery above or below the site of injury it is removed with the balloon catheter (Fogarty), see Fig. 6.1.

At the end of the operation the wound is closed with a suction drain.

Post-operative Observations and Management

The patient is put onto a broad spectrum antibiotic as infection in a wound with an artery anastomosis in the depths could result in a secondary haemorrhage. As far as the artery injury is concerned observations are made concerning two points.

1. RESTORATION OF CIRCULATION. The observations are concerned with the return of function resulting from restoration of the circulation. Sensation and muscle function should return after the operation, although if there has been much delay the return of sensation may take several days. The foot should be warm and of normal colour. Many of these patients are young men who have had accidents involving motor cycles. They have otherwise normal arteries and it should be possible to feel the foot pulses soon after the operation. As with all arterial reconstructions the pulse volume recordings give the best assessment of the success of the repair.

2. HAEMORRHAGE. Local swelling and excessive drainage from the suction drain may indicate bleeding from the suture line, and in some instances the patient may have to be returned to the theatre.

21
Angioma

The term angioma suggests that the lesion is a tumour of blood vessels. However, the term is merely descriptive and angiomas are not true tumours but malformations like other congenital deformities. There are a number of different types which have typical clinical appearances and characteristic natural history.

Strawberry Angioma

The strawberry angioma is sometimes called a strawberry naevus using the word naevus as meaning birth mark. This is not strictly true as the strawberry angioma is rarely present at birth but appears when the baby is a few weeks old. It first appears as a red mark on the skin which increases rapidly in size for some months to form a swelling resembling the colour of a ripe strawberry. When these lesions appear they are of great concern to the baby's mother. This is particularly so when the angioma appears on the face including the mouth or eyelid.

The behaviour of the strawberry naevus is very characteristic. After an initial spurt of growth it tends to grow slowly with the child until the child is about 5 or 6 years old. It then begins to blanch in the centre and gradually to regress. It eventually disappears without trace.

During the period of growth the mother is always very anxious and usually presses for active treatment. Many treatments have been used but all forms of treatment are inclined to leave some sort of scar, and the best result is obtained by leaving the angioma alone and awaiting natural regression.

Port Wine Stain

The port wine stain is present at birth and is a much more serious and difficult problem.

The skin comprises two parts. The superficial half, which is called the epidermis, is continually changing as the superficial cells fall off to be replaced by cells from below. The deep half of the skin is a fibro-elastic layer which is permanent and unchanging. The port wine stain is a malformation of small blood vessels in this layer of the skin which causes it to be of a dull blue or purple colour. Unfortunately it often affects the face or neck and is cosmetically very unsightly. Also there is no tendency for the port wine stain to regress and it grows steadily with the patient.

Treatment

Treatment of port wine stains is very difficult. Radiotherapy has been used but the results are disappointing and sometimes disastrous so that this form of treatment is now never used. Radiation has a patchy effect on the blood vessels of the angioma causing a patchy blue and white result which is not a cosmetic improvement. If radiation is used on the face of a growing child it may affect and retard the growth of the bones of the face, causing a much more serious deformity.

Excision followed by suture or grafting of the defect may be used, but extensive grafts on the face tend to scar or to look unsightly and the cosmetic result is again disappointing.

Probably the best form of treatment is the use of cosmetics to cover the discolouration.

Cavernous Angioma

The cavernous angioma is also present at birth and is a malformation of veins giving rise to a blue lump which may be compressible if it consists mainly of blood inside veins. In other cases there is quite a lot of fibrous tissue in the cavernous angioma which does not compress.

The cavernous angioma may occur superficially when it involves the skin and subcutaneous tissue. This type of angioma may also occur in the viscera. The liver is a common site but it very rarely gives rise to symptoms and is usually a chance finding at autopsy. A more serious but rare site of a cavernous angioma is the small intestine. Such an angioma may give rise to intestinal bleeding, but the diagnosis is rarely made before an exploratory laparotomy for gastro-intestinal bleeding.

Treatment

Cavernous angiomas are usually amenable to surgical treatment, and if cosmetically troublesome they should be excised. Although blood vessels are usually thrombosed by radiation this form of treatment is very undesirable in a child. Apart from the danger of inhibiting growth which has already been mentioned there is a risk of late malignant change in skin which has been irradiated. It is a good rule to say that radiation should never be used other than for malignant conditions.

Multiple Telangiectasis

This is a rare familial condition in which there are multiple capillary angiomata each about 1–3 mm in diameter. The condition may be diagnosed by seeing the small red spots inside the mouth but they in fact extend throughout the stomach and small intestine. The importance of the condition is that the stomach and intestinal lesions may bleed giving rise to chronic anaemia.

The lesions are too many for surgical treatment but most cases can be kept in reasonable health by supplementing the intake of iron.

Congenital Arteriovenous Fistulae

In this condition, which is usually confined to a limb, there is widespread malformation of the arteries and veins. The main abnormality is that there are multiple minute connections throughout the limb between the small arteries and veins. Often there is a port wine stain in part of the overlying skin. The arteriovenous connection has the effect of greatly increasing the flow of blood in the leg and this causes the limb to grow more than the normal leg. This growth is not only in girth but also in length in consequence of the increased blood flow to the growing part of the bone which is called the epiphysis.

In the more severe and extensive types of arteriovenous fistula there is an increase in the output of blood from the heart. After many years this may cause enlargement of the heart and rarely heart failure.

The condition is always very widespread and no treatment is possible.

Part 2

Surgery of The Peripheral Veins

22
Anatomy and Physiology of the Venous System in the Leg

Blood reaches the capillaries of the leg through the arterial system and is then collected in the veins for return to the right side of the heart. There are three groups of veins to be considered:

1. The Superficial Veins (Fig. 22.1)

The superficial veins run in the subcutaneous fat and are usually visible through the skin. Most of the veins including those on the dorsum of the foot drain into the long saphenous vein. This vein begins on the dorsum of the foot and runs on the front of the medial malleolus of the ankle where it is sometimes used for intravenous therapy. It then runs the full length of the leg receiving tributaries from the superficial veins of the leg and thigh and terminates by joining the main femoral vein at the top of the thigh just below the inguinal ligament.

The short saphenous vein runs from the foot behind the lateral malleolus and up the middle of the back of the leg and terminates by joining the popliteal vein behind the knee.

All the superficial veins have valves which prevent the reflux of blood in a distal direction.

2. Deep Veins (Fig. 22.2)

The deep system of veins run with the named arteries in the leg (Fig. 22.2). They are usually multiple and there are two or three veins accompanying each artery, the peroneal, posterior tibial and anterior tibial. These veins are individually quite small compared with the superficial veins and also have valves to encourage the flow of blood towards the heart. At the level of the knee the accompanying veins join to form a large vessel, the popliteal vein, which continues in the thigh where it runs with the femoral artery and is called the femoral vein. At the top of the thigh it is joined by the deep femoral vein to form the common femoral vein, which continues in the pelvis as the external and then the common iliac vein to reach the interior vena cava, where it is joined by its fellow from the opposite side.

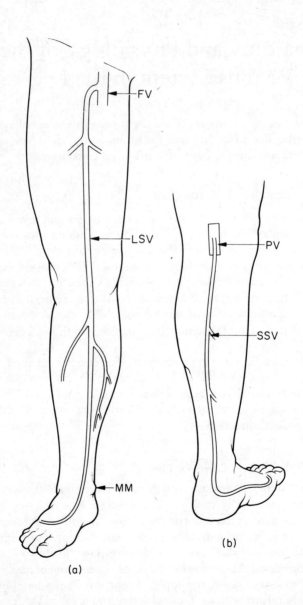

(a)

(b)

Fig. 22.1 Normal superficial veins, (a) anterior and (b) posterior. FV, femoral vein; LSV, long saphenous vein; PV, popliteal vein; SSV, short saphenous vein; MM, medial malleolus.

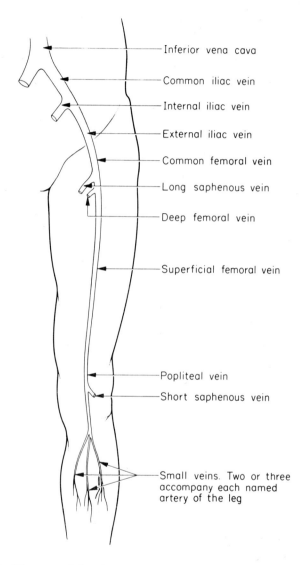

Inferior vena cava

Common iliac vein

Internal iliac vein

External iliac vein

Common femoral vein

Long saphenous vein

Deep femoral vein

Superficial femoral vein

Popliteal vein

Short saphenous vein

Small veins. Two or three accompany each named artery of the leg

Fig. 22.2 The normal distribution of the deep veins in the leg.

3. Communicating Veins

These veins join the deep and superficial system and they have particular importance. They are sometimes called perforating veins. When the communicating veins are not functioning properly serious trouble may arise in the leg. Two communications have already been mentioned. These are the termination of the long saphenous vein where it joins the femoral vein, and the termination of the short saphenous vein in the popliteal vein. There are usually a number of other communications but the exact site is variable. There is usually a communicator between the long saphenous vein and the femoral vein at the lower third of the thigh, and a number of others between the long saphenous or its main branches and the deep veins below the knee.

Physiology of the Venous Return

There is a pressure of 12 mm of mercury at the venous end of the capillary and this pressure is responsible for the continued flow of blood into the veins. There is a gradual pressure gradient from that in the left ventricle of the heart to the right atrium which is the basic cause of the continued flow of blood in the correct direction. This is sometimes called *vis a tergo* of 'force from behind'. The position of the leg does not affect the flow. Of course when the leg is down as in the erect posture, the venous pressure is equal to that due to pressure from behind (12 mm mercury) plus the hydrostatic pressure, but the arterial pressure is also raised by the same hydrostatic pressure so that the hydrostatic effect on the venous and arterial sides is equal and the effect is neutralized. However, experience shows that gravity does have a small effect and when there is arterial occlusion the capillary circulation is improved if the leg is lowered.

At rest the pressures in the deep and superficial veins have been shown to be identical, but with exercise there is a sharp rise in the pressure in the deep veins. This is caused by compression of the tissues of the leg by contraction of the muscles. When the pressure in the deep veins rises, the blood is propelled proximally towards the heart because the valves prevent flow in the opposite direction. In addition the communicating veins possess valves which prevent reflux from the deep to the superficial system through the communicators. The sudden drop in pressure in the deep veins which accompanies the cessation of exercise causes blood to flow into the deep veins from the superficial veins so that the whole of the superficial system drains into the deep system, and provided the valves are fully competent the blood never flows out from the deep to the superficial veins. This mechanism is an important contribution to the return of blood from the leg, and is called the calf (or venous) pump (Fig. 22.3).

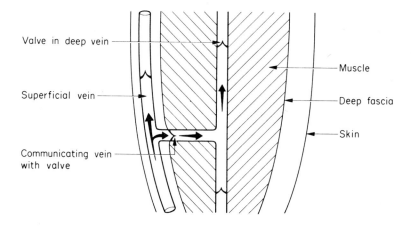

Fig. 22.3 Diagrammatic representation of the calf pump. The normal direction of flow in communicating veins is indicated by the arrows.

23
Varicose Veins

Varicose veins are dilated, tortuous and lengthened superficial veins. Once the veins are dilated the valves become incompetent as they do not reach across the dilated vein, and the pressure in the vein increases, so gradually causing the varicosities to increase.

Uncomplicated varicose veins cause few symptoms. They are far more common in women and treatment is often sought because of the unsightly appearance. In addition there is no doubt that they cause some pain, particularly after a period of standing.

Predisposing Factors

1. The most important predisposing cause of varicose veins is compression of the main veins in the pelvis. The most common cause of this is pregnancy, and many women suffer from varicose veins during pregnancy which tend to regress or disappear after delivery.
2. In other cases there is no known cause but simply a constitutional tendency to varicose veins. In some cases the valves on the perforating veins are incompetent so that blood escapes from the deep veins during walking and causes local varicosities. The most common valve incompetence responsible for varicose veins is that guarding the entrance of the long saphenous vein into the femoral and the short saphenous vein into the popliteal vein. When these valves are incompetent there is dilation of the main saphenous trunks, and their tributaries become incompetent (Fig. 23.1).
3. A rare cause is congenital arteriovenous fistula. In this condition the child is born with a deformity of the blood vessels of the leg in which there are multiple communications between the small arteries and veins, and this gives rise to raised pressure in the venous system. As a result the veins tend to become varicose. To a surgeon the condition is important as a cause of varicose veins in childhood or adolescence. No treatment can be directed to the varicose veins.

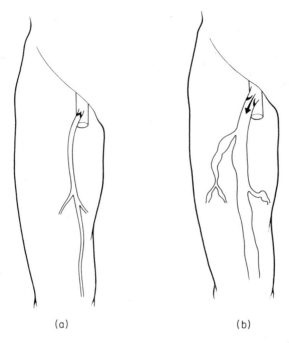

Fig. 23.1 (a) Normal drainage of long saphenous vein into femoral vein with competent valve. (b) Incompetent valve causing reflux and varicose veins.

Complications of Varicose Veins

1. Oedema of the Ankles

The increased hydrostatic pressure in the capillaries resulting from the stagnant flow of blood in varicose veins may cause a little oedema. It is important to remember that anything more than trivial oedema is likely to be caused by pathological changes in the deep or communicating veins.

2. Superficial Thrombophlebitis

Any varicose veins may without warning become inflamed and thrombosed. The vein in question becomes very painful and walking is difficult. Examination shows the vein to be hard because of thrombosis, and red and tender because of the inflammation in its wall. Treatment consists of rest until the pain subsides, and most surgeons try to assist the process by the use of an anti-inflammatory drug such as Butazolidine. This drug may cause or exacerbate gastroduodenal ulceration so that it should always be taken on a full stomach, and the presence of gastric or duodenal ulceration is an absolute contra-indication.

3. Venous Eczema

Eczema is a generalized condition of the skin but it is inclined to be more severe in a leg with varicose veins, and leg eczema may be improved by treatment of the varicose veins in the leg. However, it must be emphasized that varicose veins are not the basic cause of eczema and it may recur after adequate treatment of the varicose veins.

4. Ulcers

Leg ulcers are not usually a complication of simple varicose veins but of other abnormalities in the venous circulation and should properly be called venous ulcers and not varicose ulcers. Occasionally, however, a patient with uncomplicated varicose veins may develop a typical ulcer.

5. Bleeding

Sudden and severe bleeding may occur as a result of rupture of a varicose vein. The immediate first aid treatment is to raise the leg to empty blood from the veins and to apply external pressure over the bleeding point. Later the vein should be excised.

Treatment of Uncomplicated Varicose Veins

Fashion and shortage of in-patient facilities for surgical treatment account for the many changes in the treatment of uncomplicated varicose veins which have occurred in the past 50 years. Some surgeons treat all cases with injections and others by surgery; some treat only the more severe cases surgically.

A new factor has emerged in recent years. The long saphenous vein may be required as a graft to the femoral artery in cases of leg ischaemia. It can also be used as a graft for cases of coronary artery occlusion. This makes it imperative to conserve the long saphenous vein whenever possible.

Injection Treatment of Varicose Veins with Sclerosant Substance

For many years the most commonly used sclerosant was 5% ethanolamine oleate which acted by irritating and damaging the intima of the vein causing a localized thrombosis. In this technique the surgeon introduced a needle into the varicose vein with the patient standing and the vein full. The injection was given into the full vein without moving the patient from the standing position. The resulting thrombosis was often painful and extended for a considerable distance beyond the site of injection. Although initially quite satisfactory, this technique had the disadvantage that the thrombosed area tended to recanalize with recurrence of the varicosities. This technique is not now used and ethanolamine is no longer manufactured.

Empty Vein Technique of Injecting Varicose Veins (Compression Sclerotherapy)

In this technique the needle is also introduced into the vein when it is full. This condition can be achieved by standing the patient but it is more convenient to use a venous tourniquet with the patient lying down. Once the needle is inserted the vein is emptied by removing the tourniquet and elevating the leg. The injection is then given into the empty vein with the object of causing irritation of its wall which will stick together instead of causing a thrombus. In this technique 1 ml of sodium tetradecyl sulphate (STD) is used. To further encourage the process a foam pad is placed over the vein and kept in position with a bandage and an elastic stocking. As some patients show skin sensitivity to the foam pad, a layer of bandage should be applied to the skin before putting the foam pad in position. This external compression must be kept up for 6 weeks, both night and day, and at the end of this period the varicose vein should be converted to a fibrous cord which cannot recanalize to cause a recurrence. The process may be likened to the use of glue on woodwork in which compression is required to get adhesion of two surfaces. There is some risk of thrombosis at the site of injection and this may spread through a communicating vein to the deep system causing a deep vein thrombosis and possibly a pulmonary embolism. To avoid this the patient is asked to walk at least two miles a day to keep a good flow of blood in the deep veins.

It is known that patients taking the contraceptive pill may develop a deep vein thrombosis, and it is wise to stop taking the contraceptive pill during treatment.

This type of treatment is performed on an outpatient basis and this is its main advantage. It is, however, a rather difficult technique and is quite unsuitable for use in a hot climate as the use of compression bandages and elastic stockings would be unbearable.

Surgical Treatment

The main objects of surgical treatment are to eliminate any incompetent perforating veins and to excise varicosities which may not regress after ligation of the perforators.

Saphenous Vein Stripping Operation

This operation can be performed on the long or short saphenous veins depending on the surgeon's interpretation of the origin of the varicosities in the leg. It must be emphasized, however, that the saphenous vein should not be excised unless it is considered abnormally dilated, as its later need in cardiac or vascular surgery cannot be anticipated.

The steps in the operation of stripping the long saphenous vein are illustrated in Fig. 23.2.

1. The long saphenous vein is explored at the groin, and ligatured and divided close to its connection with the femoral vein.
2. The long saphenous vein is identified through a small incision at the ankle just in front of the medial malleolus. The vein is then divided and the lower end ligated. The wire stripper is inserted into the proximal end of the divided vein and threaded up the vein until it emerges in the saphenous vein previously exposed in the groin.
3. The vein is securely tied just above the acorn on the stripper at the ankle.
4. A handle is fixed to the stripper wire where it has appeared at the groin to enable the surgeon to pull the whole vein out from the ankle to the groin.
5. As the vein is stripped all the varicose tributaries are torn off and some bleeding into the subcutaneous tissue of the leg is

inevitable. To minimize bleeding the table is tilted about 35–40° to empty the veins, and a firm supporting bandage is applied to the leg as the vein is stripped.

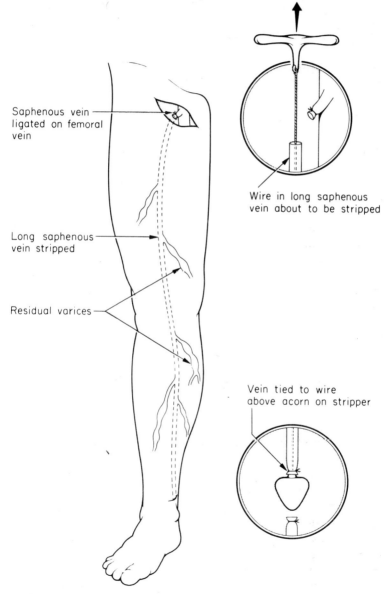

Fig. 23.2   Operation of stripping long saphenous vein.

Sapheno-femoral Ligation

This operation is sometimes known as Trendelenburg's operation.

It is an essential step in the treatment of varicose veins when there is incompetence and retrograde flow at the sapheno-femoral junction. In these cases the saphenous vein is felt in the groin and is considerably above the normal calibre. In addition there is an impulse or thrill over the vein at the groin when the patient coughs.

The operation simply consists of exposing the junction of the saphenous and femoral veins at the groin, and ligating and dividing the long saphenous vein flush with the femoral vein.

Multiple Excisions

Multiple excisions may be performed alone or in combination with sapheno-femoral ligation. In this operation it is essential to mark the varices with ink accurately before the operation as they cannot always be seen once the patient is on the operating table and the varices emptied of blood.

In the modern operation 3 mm incisions are made with a No. 11 scalpel blade over the varices and in the positions marked before the operation. At each tiny incision it is possible to identify and tease out with fine instruments several centimetres of varicose vein. At the completion these incisions are closed with micropore tape. Sutures are unnecessary. A compression bandage is applied on the operating table.

Post-operative Observations on Operations for Varicose Veins

In the immediate post-operative period the foot should be inspected to ensure that its circulation is not endangered by an elastic bandage which has been too tightly applied in the operating room. Any change in colour of the foot should be reported to the surgeon, and if there is doubt concerning the circulation the elastic bandage must be removed.

The main later risk of operations for veins is that of a deep vein thrombosis which may be followed by pulmonary embolus. To avoid this the patient is got out of bed on the first day and made to walk. When resting the leg should be kept with the knee straight and elevated on a stool to promote a good flow of blood in the deep veins.

The patient may be discharged in 48 hours and will need to be seen on the seventh day for removal of sutures and support bandages. A light support may then be applied for a further seven days.

Surgical treatment has the advantage to the patient that it is quickly over and that the results are more certain than those of any form of injection. However, the need for a hospital bed is a serious drawback in some communities.

24
Chronic Venous Insufficiency in the Leg

This condition is responsible for a great deal of pain, suffering and chronic disability. The main problem is a difficulty in effecting an adequate flow of venous blood through the leg. It is due to partial obstruction of the deep veins by thrombus, or to incompetent valves in the deep veins. In each case there is a difficulty in effecting venous return, particularly with the patient in the upright position when clear veins with adequate valves are essential if the calf pump is to operate successfully. Incompetence of the perforating veins causes similar but less severe symptoms. In most cases there is a history suggesting that a deep vein thrombosis has been present in the past. The natural history of a deep vein thrombosis is that it will gradually recanalize. However, when such a vein recanalizes the valves are damaged and permanently incompetent, giving rise to the condition of chronic venous insufficiency.

When a patient with normal veins stands or walks, there is a flow of blood from the superficial to the deep veins through the perforators. There is also a good centrally directed flow in the deep veins as a result of the functions of the valves which protect the communicators and which are present in the deep veins (page 120).

When the valves are damaged or destroyed, the normal flow of blood is interfered with (Fig. 24.1). Proximal flow in the deep veins is reduced and there is a flow out through the communicating veins to the superficial veins. This difficulty with removal of blood from the leg causes a feeling of bursting, and there is swelling of the leg particularly in its lower part.

The flow of blood into the superficial veins causes a high pressure in the superficial veins and capillaries in the region of the ankle, so reducing flow and tissue nutrition. The fatty tissues may undergo necrosis and form a hard woody mass. Later the overlying skin necroses to form a venous ulcer.

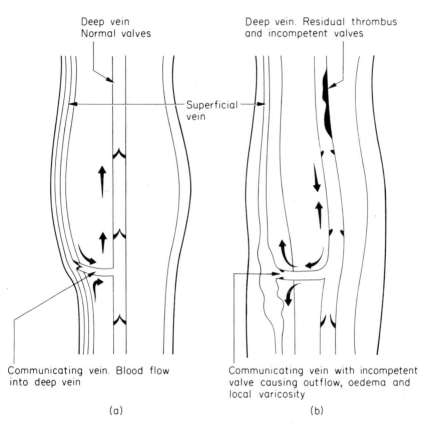

Fig. 24.1 Post-thombotic leg to illustrate cause of chronic venous insufficiency: (a) normal; (b) post-phlebitic.

Clinical Appearance of the Leg

The leg shows a variable amount of oedema. The skin may be ulcerated and there is extensive brown pigmentation of the skin. This is derived from blood pigments which leave the capillaries because of the high pressure in the veins and capillaries. Varicose veins are notably absent or minimally present. If they are present, varicose veins are usually situated in a localized area in the region of the perforators.

Treatment of Venous Insufficiency

Prevention

This serious disability results in most cases from a deep vein thrombosis. All of those who look after sick people have a duty constantly to strive to avoid this complication of medical or surgical treatment. In addition, once a deep vein thrombosis has been diagnosed the strongest measures should be taken to arrest its progress and, if practicable, to disperse the thrombus.

Conservative Treatment

Elevation

In many cases the only practical measures are conservative. The patient suffering from chronic venous insufficiency will have to adapt to a new way of life. Walking is not likely to be harmful but the patient should never stand still when he can sit. When sitting the leg must be elevated, and the patient should spend as much time as possible sitting down with the leg elevated above the horizontal. In this position the blood flows easily back to the heart and the high venous pressure at the ankle is relieved.

Bandaging

The object of bandaging is to prevent the reflux of blood through the communicating veins. If the position of the perforator can be located a foam pad is placed at this point and secured in position with an elastic or elastocrepe bandage. A support or elastic stocking is also worn for extra support. If the patient walks while wearing this external support the superficial veins are compressed and the outpouring of blood through the perforating vein is prevented, so encouraging the venous return along its proper channel—the deep venous system.

Treatment of Venous Ulcers

There are two aspects to the treatment of venous ulcers:

1. To Eliminate Infection

A variety of local applications may be used. In spite of the use of many modern agents Eusol remains a very useful local application. If mixed with liquid paraffin the difficulty and discomfort of the sticking dressing is eliminated. A culture should be taken and may indicate the need for some special local treatment or a systemic antibiotic.

2. To Restore Normal Physiology

In severe and long-standing ulcers, the quickest way to restore the venous return and initiate healing is to put the patient to bed with the foot of the bed elevated on blocks. Venous return is at once normal and the conditions are set for healing of the ulcer. At rest in bed healing is usually rapid.

In patients who have less severe signs of venous insufficiency and a small area of ulceration ambulant treatment may be attempted. The same two principles of treatment must be observed. The ulcer is treated with an antiseptic such as Eusol, and external pressure applied to prevent blood reflux through the perforators. One effective technique is to apply a paste dressing which sets to give a firm support. The patient can have the ulcer inspected and the paste support reapplied at weekly intervals. If progress is good the treatment is continued, but if the ulcer fails to show signs of healing the patient must be advised to come into hospital for bed rest and elevation.

Venous ulcers are usually easy to treat but there is a high incidence of recurrence if the patient returns to normal life without an external support. Once a patient has had an ulcer she needs external support in the form of a plastic pad and elastic stockings for the rest of her life.

Surgical Treatment of Venous Insufficiency

Surgery does not play a very important part but is indicated when conservative measures fail. The object of surgical treatment is to ligate and divide the perforators which are a main cause of the trouble.

Phlebography

Before embarking on surgical treatment the patient should be X-rayed to locate the sites of perforating veins.

The patient is placed on the X-ray table and a cannula is placed in a vein on the foot. If an injection of radio-opaque dye is given into a superficial vein on the foot it will pass straight up the superficial saphenous venous system. To prevent this a venous tourniquet is applied just above the ankle. This directs the dye through the communicating veins at this level to the deep veins where it passes proximally. When the dye reaches incompetent perforating veins in the leg they can be clearly seen and recorded by taking radiographs.

Operation

Two routes are available. In the anterior approach the incision is made behind the subcutaneous border of the tibia. This approach has the disadvantage that healing is sometimes very slow.

An alternative incision is down the middle of the back of the leg, the seam of stocking incision. Once through the deep fascia the superficial layers can be dissected away until the perforators are identified and ligated. The wound is closed with interrupted sutures to the skin.

Post-operative Management

The leg is best kept elevated with blocks under the foot of the bed to minimize swelling. The patient should be ambulant on the first day but when not walking the leg should be kept elevated. There is always a tendency for the limb to swell, and recurrent ulcer is a possibility so that most patients are given an elastic stocking to wear permanently. The seam of stocking incisions heal slowly and sutures should not be removed before the tenth day at the earliest.

25
Thromboembolism: (1) Vein Thrombosis

The importance of vein thrombosis is twofold. The thrombus may become detached from the vein in which it has formed to be swept into the venous circulation to cause a pulmonary embolus which may be fatal. Secondly, if the thrombus remains in the site in which it has formed it will obstruct the venous return from the leg and may cause serious disability from chronic venous insufficiency. Vein thrombosis is a well-known complication of surgery. It also occurs in patients in medical wards and may occur spontaneously in patients as a primary disease.

Common Sites of Vein Thrombosis

We are only concerned with thrombi forming in the deep veins. Thrombosis in superficial veins complicated by inflammation (thrombophlebitis) rarely causes any serious trouble unless the thrombosis extends through a perforator to involve the deep veins.

1. Iliac Vein Thrombosis

This is particularly a complication of pregnancy and pelvic operations but may follow any other form of surgery. A feature of all thrombi which form in veins is their loose attachment to the wall of the vein (Fig. 25.1). Venography often shows that the thrombus has a very small area of attachment to the vein wall. The rest of the thrombus floats like an eel in the blood stream. This accounts for the fact that in many cases the circulation is not sufficiently obstructed by the thrombus to give rise to any clinical signs. The second result is the ease of detachment to form an embolus which may be the first sign that a vein thrombosis has occurred.

In other cases of iliac vein thrombosis the occlusion is complete. As the common and external iliac veins are the final pathway for all blood from the leg the sudden and complete closure of these veins

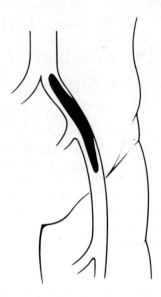

Fig. 25.1 Iliac vein thrombosis. Note narrow base of attachment to iliac vein wall and incomplete obstruction to blood flow.

gives rise to dramatic symptoms. The whole leg suddenly becomes very swollen and white in colour. Clinically this is known as a 'white leg' and is characteristic of an iliac vein thrombosis.

Prognosis of Iliac Vein Thrombosis

If the iliac vein remains permanently occluded the patient will suffer from the symptoms of chronic venous insufficiency comprising swelling of the leg and a bursting pain on walking. However, because the leg veins and perforators have not been involved with thrombus their valves usually remain competent so that the patient does not suffer from leg ulceration. More often an iliac vein containing a thrombus undergoes gradual recanalization, and there is often a negligible disability one year after the event.

2. Calf Vein and Femoropopliteal Vein Thrombosis

Thrombosis often begins in the small veins of the calf muscles, or in cusps of valves in the popliteal and femoral veins. Once the process begins it tends to spread. However, the veins are not often completely occluded so that there is a good flow of blood and no signs of venous obstruction. The loose attachment of thrombus to the vein wall is the cause of sudden and unexpected embolism.

Diagnosis of Deep Vein Thrombosis

Diagnosis of a deep vein thrombosis is one of the most difficult things in surgery. It has been estimated that only 20% of deep vein thromboses are diagnosed before an embolism takes place. It therefore follows that in the majority of cases there are no physical signs and the diagnosis cannot be made on clinical grounds. Some signs may be present.

1. Pyrexia. A low fever is sometimes present. If the patient has a low fever which cannot be explained on other grounds it may be the only sign of a vein thrombosis.

2. Calf Tenderness. Tenderness in the calf is often present when the calf veins are thrombosed. Unfortunately calf tenderness does not always mean that a calf vein thrombosis is present.

3. There may in a few cases be other signs such as swelling of the leg and dilatation of the superficial veins. Warmth is also a characteristic feature and the limb should be carefully compared with its fellow.

Diagnostic Aids

As so many patients with a calf vein thrombosis have no clinical signs it is necessary to investigate every post-operative case if the diagnosis is to be made before an embolism occurs. Most surgeons do not practise these tests routinely but for the sake of completeness they are described.

1. Venography. In suspicious cases venography may be performed. This gives the most reliable information concerning the presence of thrombosis in the deep veins, but it is an invasive technique and not entirely without risk. Another difficulty concerns the amount of time needed in the X-ray department. No X-ray department could cope with the routine venography on all post-operative cases.

2. Isotope Studies. Human fibrinogen labelled with radioactive iodine (^{125}I) is used for this test. This is injected and the legs tested for radioactivity two hours later. Fibrinogen is present in the formation of thrombus and the test is positive when there is recent thrombosis. The test is unreliable in the thigh and pelvis but correlation with venography shows a high degree of accuracy. Unfortunately the technique is complicated and unsuitable for routine use.

3. Doppler Ultrasound Technique. The Doppler effect is more familiar in audible sound. The principle depends on the fact that the sound of a passing object, such as a railway train whistle, drops in pitch as it passes.

In the ultrasound technique a beam of ultrasound is directed at the venous flow. When the beam encounters a column of moving blood cells it is reflected causing an alteration in the frequency of the beam which can be amplified to drive a loud speaker. This is an easy test for routine use but it does not distinguish between a recent and an old venous occlusion (see also p. 18).

Prevention of Vein Thrombosis

Much work has been concentrated on efforts to prevent vein thrombosis especially as it occurs after routine surgical operations. Unfortunately there is still no clear indication that any particular form of prophylaxis is worth using as a routine measure.

1. External Support. Bandages have been used for this purpose, and more recently elastic stockings which are specially made to give a gradation of pressure from the foot to the thigh. A pressure gradient of 18 to 8 mm of mercury is recommended, and it has been shown that this considerably increases the flow of blood in the femoral vein. There is some evidence that the incidence of vein thrombosis and pulmonary embolism is reduced but accurate fitting of elastic stockings to each pre-operative patient would be a very large and expensive task.

2. Anticoagulants. Anticoagulants have been used for many years, but the use of Heparin or coumarin drugs has been unpopular because of the high incidence of haemorrhage-complicating surgery done under these conditions. Recently a regime of low-dose heparin has been on trial which is reported to give a lowered incidence of vein thrombosis without significantly increasing the rate of haematoma and haemorrhage. In this regime the patients are given 5000 units of

Heparin by subcutaneous injection 2 hours before the operation and then 5000 units eight-hourly for seven days.

3. One of the simplest and safest measures is to raise the foot of the bed with blocks to encourage a rapid venous circulation.

Measures Taken During Surgery

It has been assumed that the immobility of the calf muscles during an operation under general anaesthetic contributes to the incidence of thrombosis. A variety of measures have been tried during surgery but there is no evidence that any of these contribute significantly to a lowered incidence of thrombosis.

1. A commonly employed technique is to put a small pillow under the heels to raise the calves of the legs from the table, so removing pressure which might cause some stagnation of blood flow.
2. An electrical device to cause repeated contractions of the calf muscle during surgery.
3. An appliance which is fitted round the leg and which contracts regularly in an attempt to mimic the effects of the calf pump which normally operates when the patient is walking.

Treatment of Venous Thrombosis

Bed Rest

Patients with a deep vein thrombosis are always treated by bed rest. It is obvious that any movement may dislodge a thrombus and cause a pulmonary embolus so the patient is kept at rest in the hope that the thrombus will adhere firmly to the vein wall. Surgeons keep patients in bed for variable times after diagnosing a vein thrombosis but an average time is seven days. Many surgeons ask for the foot of the bed to be raised to help the venous return, and bandage the leg to divert blood from the superficial veins, so increasing the flow in the deep veins.

Anticoagulants

The object of anticoagulant treatment is to stop any spread of the thrombosis which is already present. Anticoagulants do not dissolve clot which is already present and the long-term effects of venous insufficiency are not reduced. However, further thrombosis is prevented and embolism made less likely.

Normal Coagulation of Blood

The normal process of coagulation of the blood is a very complicated biochemical reaction. Blood consists of a liquid—plasma—in which are floating and circulating the red and white blood cells. The plasma contains a substance called fibrinogen which is converted to a clot called fibrin. In the earlier phase of the clotting process a substance called thrombin is formed in the blood, and it is the action of thrombin on fibrinogen which gives rise to fibrin.

Prothrombin → Thrombin + Fibrinogen → Fibrin

Heparinization

Heparin is given intravenously and has an immediate anticoagulant effect. The usual regime is to give a dose of 5000 international units intravenously, and then to give 20 000 international units every 12 hours by slow intravenous drip. It is most convenient to do this with an automatic syringe which is emptied with a clockwork mechanism in 12 hours.

Short periods of heparinization do not require laboratory control, but if the heparinization is prolonged more than 72 hours then it is wise to do the plasma clotting time (PCT) every day. In this test the patient's plasma and a control plasma are each treated by the addition of thrombin. The normal plasma clots as a result of the action of thrombin on fibrinogen in the plasma giving rise to fibrin. Heparin inhibits the action of thrombin so that the patient's heparinized plasma will take longer to clot. It is best to keep the plasma clotting time at between two and three times normal.

Warfarin

Warfarin is the usual form of oral anticoagulant in use. Vitamin K acts as a catalyst in the formation of thrombin. Warfarin prevents the formation of Vitamin K in the liver and so slows down the formation of the thrombin which is necessary for conversion of fibrinogen to fibrin. The advantage of Warfarin is that it can be given by mouth. It takes about 48 hours to become effective so that it must be combined with Heparin if an immediate effect is required.

The immediate dose is 30 mg, and it is usual to estimate pro-thrombin time after 48 hours. Subsequent doses are based on the daily prothrombin time but a dose of 5–10 mg daily is usual.

Streptokinase

Streptokinase activates substances in recent clot called fibrinolysins whose function it is to dissolve a thrombus. If treatment with Strep-tokinase is successful the thrombus disappears and the vein returns to normal.

Streptokinase operates in a similar way on thrombus which is sealing a recent surgical incision and if it is used within ten days of an operation serious haemorrhage is likely. Recent surgery is an absolute contra-indication to the use of Streptokinase. It is also contra-indicated after such investigations as lumbar puncture and arteriography, and in patients with peptic ulcers or other lesions which might bleed. Streptokinase and Heparin must not be given at the same time.

It is usual to control the use of Streptokinase by doing a venogram before and after treatment. Many patients show anaphylactic reactions following the injection of Streptokinase and to prevent this they are given Prednisolone.

Streptokinase Treatment Regime

1. Prednisolone 25 mg orally before treatment and twice daily during treatment.
2. A loading dose of 600 000 international units of Streptokin-ase is given intravenously.
3. Streptokinase is then given in a 5% glucose solution at the rate of 100 000 international units per hour. It is usual to continue the treatment for 3–5 days.
4. When Streptokinase treatment is stopped there is a tendency for re-thrombosis to occur and therefore the patient is started on Heparin and later oral anticoagulants.

Antidote to Streptokinase

If the patient suffers an acute haemorrhage while being treated with Streptokinase the treatment must be stopped at once. The anti-fibrinolytic agent which is used as an antidote is aminocaproic acid. This drug must be available if Streptokinase treatment is used.

Thrombectomy

An alternative technique for removal of thrombus and for restoring the veins to normal is to remove the thrombus by an operation called thrombectomy. This operation is not often done because many surgeons believe that recurrence of the thrombus is likely after its removal. Thrombectomy may be recommended:

1. When the thrombosis occurs too soon after the operation for the safe use of Streptokinase.
2. When large vessels such as the iliac and femoral veins are involved causing a white leg.

Operation of Thrombectomy

The operation can be performed under a local anaesthetic. The femoral vein in the groin is dissected and handled with care so that the thrombus inside is not dislodged. The technique is to pass a balloon catheter through the thrombus, to inflate the balloon, and to withdraw the inflated balloon so extracting the thrombus. The technique is similar to that shown in Fig. 6.1 which illustrates the use of a balloon catheter for removal of an aortic embolus.

Following this operation the patient must be treated with anticoagulants to prevent recurrent thrombosis.

Post-operative Observations

Sometimes these patients are treated with anticoagulants throughout the operative and post-operative period because of the risk of recurrent thrombosis.

Observations must therefore be particularly directed to the operation site so that any signs of bleeding can be noted. There may be external bleeding into the dressings or internal bleeding causing a large haematoma. The wound should be inspected at 15-minute intervals in the recovery room and less frequently when back in the ward.

26

Thromboembolism: (2) Pulmonary Embolism

When a thrombus forms in a leg vein there is always a risk that it will become detached from its point of origin and be swept in the great veins to the heart (Fig. 26.1). It reaches the right atrium, passes through the tricuspid valve to enter the right ventricle, and then leaves the heart through the pulmonary artery. This is called a pulmonary embolus. The effects at this point depend on the size of the embolus.

1. A small thrombus passes through the main pulmonary artery and lodges in a small branch in the right or left lung. The pulmonary circulation to the segment of lung supplied by this branch is suddenly arrested. Usually the patient complains of a sudden pain in the chest and shortness of breath. The lung undergoes changes which are called infarction. In the lung there is some flow of blood from other arteries which leaks into the air spaces and which is coughed up by the patient. Haemoptysis is a characteristic feature of pulmonary embolism. Another effect is that the pleura overlying the infarcted segment becomes roughened and inflamed, and as the two pleural surfaces move together the patient complains of pain on breathing. Pain on breathing is called pleuritic pain and is another characteristic feature of pulmonary embolism. Haemoptysis and pleuritic pain are late signs coming on about 5–7 days after the embolism.
2. The effects of a pulmonary embolus vary with the size of the embolus, and in the extreme case a very large thrombus will coil up and become arrested in the main pulmonary artery and its two main branches to the two lungs. This stops the output of blood from the right ventricle and in fact stops the circulation. The patient feels severe retrosternal pain which is partly due to coronary ischaemia as the circulation is arrested and no blood is flowing into the coronary arteries. The patient rapidly shows signs of shock and may die in a few minutes.

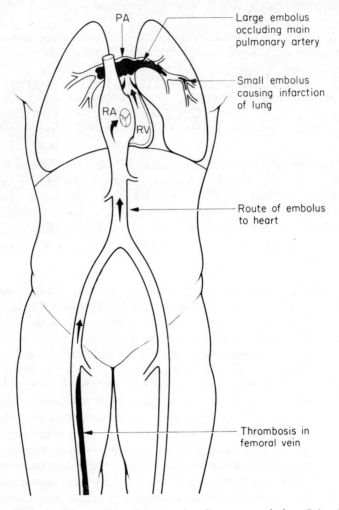

PA

Large embolus
occluding main
pulmonary artery

Small embolus
causing infarction
of lung

RA

RV

Route of embolus
to heart

Thrombosis in
femoral vein

Fig. 26.1 Deep vein thrombosis and pulmonary embolus. RA, right atrium; RV, right ventricle; PA, pulmonary artery.

3. A small non-fatal embolus may be followed by further emboli and any of these may be fatal.

Special Investigations

1. A chest X-ray is usually taken but the findings are not always characteristic, and indeed the X-ray may be normal in a patient who has a pulmonary embolus.

2. Electrocardiogram. Evidence of right heart strain is usually shown on the ECG and is due to the fact that the right ventricle is working against an obstructed pulmonary artery.

3. Radioisotope Scanning. Invasive techniques such as angiography are rarely performed as the introduction of dye into the right heart in cases of embolism is obviously risky. In isotype scanning albumen microspheres labelled with 99m technetium are injected. Subsequent scanning of the lung fields shows clear areas where the lung is infarcated by an embolus. This test is safe and reliable.

Treatment of Pulmonary Embolism

1. Anticoagulants

The patient should immediately receive full anticoagulant treatment consisting of Heparin and Warfarin as described in the treatment of vein thrombosis. The object of anticoagulation is to stop the reformation of thrombus and recurrent emboli.

2. Streptokinase

Provided the conditions mentioned in the treatment of vein thrombosis are satisfied treatment with Streptokinase can be very satisfactory. However, the patient must be more than ten days post-operative and must not have any lesion which might easily bleed. In these conditions Streptokinase may not only remove any residual thrombus in the leg but it may also cause the solution of the thrombus occluding the pulmonary artery.

3. Operations on the Vena Cava

There are some cases in which emboli are recurrent in spite of adequate treatment. Sometimes the surgical situation does not permit the use of anticoagulants because of the risk or actual complication of serious haemorrhage.

This situation is an indication to occlude the vena cava so that clots formed in the leg cannot reach the heart and lungs. The first operation done was to ligate the inferior vena cava just below the renal veins. Complete arrest of the venous circulation is usually complicated by serious disability from chronic venous insufficiency in both legs, so that surgeons have attempted to partly occlude the vena cava making openings large enough to allow the free passage of blood but too small to allow the passage of thrombus.

These operations are illustrated in Fig. 26.2 and consist of the application of an external clamp or of making a lattice of sutures across the vena cava.

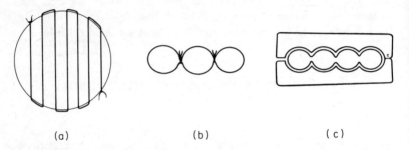

(a)   (b)   (c)

Fig. 26.2   Techniques used to prevent passage of an embolus through the inferior vena cava: (a) lattice suture; (b) suture to change lumen to three small channels; (c) external clamp to reduce size of lumen.

4. Pulmonary Embolectomy

This operation was first done by Trendelenberg in 1908. It is occasionally done today but has a high mortality. As it is difficult to predict with certainty that a patient will die of an embolus the operation is not popular with most surgeons.

Put in very simple terms the operation is an emergency one in which the heart is approached through a midline incision dividing the sternum. The pulmonary artery is opened just above the heart, the clot extracted, and the pulmonary artery sutured. In a major centre this operation can be done in the cardiac unit using cardiopulmonary bypass, but this is not essential.

Part 3

The Surgery of Portal Hypertension

27

Anatomy of Liver Circulation

Blood supply to the Liver

1. Hepatic Artery (Fig. 27.1)

The hepatic artery brings oxygenated blood to the liver. Its flow accounts for only 20% of the blood flow to the liver.

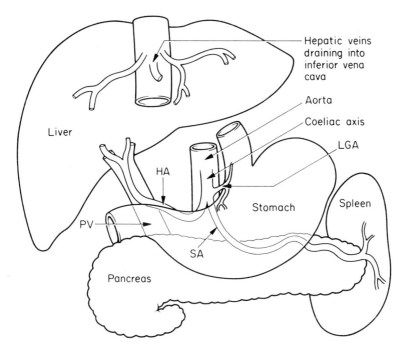

Fig. 27.1 Anatomy of the hepatic artery and hepatic veins. HA, hepatic artery; SA, splenic artery; LGA, left gastric artery; PV, portal vein.

The coeliac axis is a very large branch of the abdominal aorta. It has three large branches which are:

1. The left gastric artery which is one of the main blood vessels supplying the stomach.
2. The splenic artery which supplies the spleen.

3. The hepatic artery. This runs across the upper abdomen and divides into two main branches. These branches are the right and left branches which enter and supply oxygenated, arterial blood to the right and left lobes of the liver.

2. Portal Vein (Fig. 27.2)

The second blood vessel carrying blood to the liver is the portal vein. This carries 80% of the blood which enters the liver. The portal vein is formed by the junction of two large veins, the splenic vein which carries blood from the spleen, and the superior mesenteric vein which brings blood from the intestines. Although the portal blood is

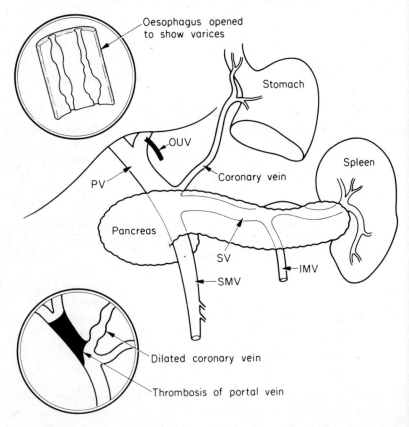

Fig. 27.2 Anatomy of the portal venous system. PV, portal vein; SV, splenic vein; SMV, superior mesenteric vein; IMV, inferior mesenteric vein; OUV, obliterated umbilical vein.

not oxygenated it is very important as it brings to the liver products of digestion which have been absorbed from the intestine.

3. Hepatic Veins (Fig. 27.1)

The hepatic artery and the portal vein together account for the blood supply to the liver. When the blood has passed through the liver it is collected into veins called the hepatic veins which are usually three or four in number and these drain into the inferior vena cava.

Functions of the Liver

The liver has many important functions. The function of the individual liver cells is dependent on the dual blood supply described above and a free drainage into the hepatic veins.

The main functions of the liver are:

1. To make bile from the blood and to collect this into tiny bile ducts within the liver. These small ducts join to form larger channels, and eventually a single duct leaves each lobe of the liver. These join to form the common bile duct which delivers bile into the duodenum.
2. The liver cells have many important functions concerned with metabolism. They also receive the products of digestion from the intestines, and foodstuffs are taken from the portal blood and altered by the liver cells to enable them to be utilized by the body or stored.
3. The liver holds about 60% of the reticulo–endothelial system. This is a system of cells distributed widely throughout the body but mainly in lymph glands, liver, spleen and bone marrow. These cells have the function of removing particulate matter such as bacteria from the blood stream.

Microanatomy of the Liver (Fig. 27.3)

The basic microanatomical structure of the liver is the liver lobule. In between the lobules are the portal tracts. These consist of a minute branch from the hepatic artery, portal vein and bile duct. These three structures are always found together in the spaces between the lobules. In the centre of the liver lobule is the hepatic vein, and these veins join together and eventually drain into the vena cava.

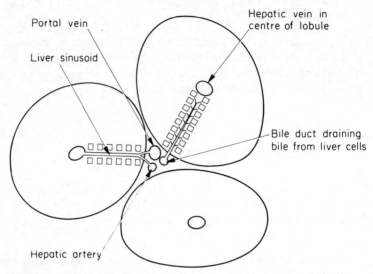

Fig. 27.3 Liver lobule and microscopic anatomy. The blood flows through the sinusoid from the portal vein and hepatic artery to the hepatic vein. In the sinusoid the blood is close to the liver cells which absorb food substances and particulate matter. Bile is discharged from the liver cells into the minute intrahepatic bile ducts.

The blood from the vessels in the portal tract runs through minute channels called sinusoids to reach the hepatic vein in the centre of the lobule. When the blood passes through the sinusoids it runs very close to the liver cells which are able to remove or add material to the blood passing through. In a similar way minute bile canaliculi receive bile from the liver cells, and the bile is received into the bile duct running in the portal tract.

28
Portal Hypertension

The normal pressure in the portal vein is 15–20 cm of saline. That is to say, if a needle connected to a tube of saline is placed in the portal vein the blood will rise about 15–20 cm in the tube. Portal hypertension is considered to be present if the pressure exceeds 25 cm of saline, but in patients who have bled from oesophageal varices the pressure is nearly always above 30 cm of saline.

Causes of Portal Hypertension

Portal hypertension will result if there is any obstruction to the flow of the portal blood. This may be at any point in the portal venous system, or there may be obstruction to the outflow of blood through the hepatic veins. Even cardiac failure will cause portal hypertension because of the raised pressure in the hepatic veins.

There are important differences in the effects which are dependent on whether the obstruction is on the portal vein side of the liver sinusoid or whether it is beyond the sinusoid. It is customary to classify cases of portal hypertension into pre-hepatic, intra-hepatic and post-hepatic causes. In the intra-hepatic group the distinction between pre- and post-sinusoidal obstruction is very important.

A. Pre-hepatic

Pre-hepatic causes are those in which the portal vein is occluded somewhere in its course before it enters the liver (Fig. 27.2).

1. Cavernous Malformation of the Portal Vein. In this condition the portal vein is replaced by a number of small veins so that although there is still some flow it is greatly reduced. Most of these cases result from umbilical infection in infancy. This spreads to give rise to an infection in the umbilical vein which has thrombosed after birth. The infection spreads into the portal vein which thromboses as a result of the infection. Later the portal vein recanalizes to give rise to multiple small channels.

2. The portal vein sometimes thromboses in cases of cirrhosis. In this case the patient may already have portal hypertension because of liver cirrhosis, and this is added to by thrombosis of the portal vein.

3. The splenic vein runs very close to the pancreas, and thrombosis of the splenic vein is a rare complication of pancreatitis. Splenic vein thrombosis may spread into the portal vein.

B. Intra-hepatic

Intra-hepatic causes of portal hypertension are those which arise within the liver itself.

1. Schistosomiasis. This is an infection by a small parasite which infects the rectum or bladder. The eggs (ova) of the parasite reach the liver in the portal blood. As the ova are foreign material to the body they cause an inflammatory reaction in and around the small tributaries of the portal vein. Later these areas of inflammation fibrose to cause a form of cirrhosis. Many patients with bilharzia also suffer from serious malnutrition and anaemia.

2. Cirrhosis—Pre-sinusoidal Obstruction. Cases of cirrhosis of the liver vary in their severity and also in their effects on the portal pressure. In cases of cirrhosis there is regeneration of liver tissue and also fibrosis. In early cases the fibrosis is limited to the portal tracts which are compressed by the fibrosis causing pre-sinusoidal obstruction. In cases of cirrhosis there may be impairment of liver function and this will complicate the management of portal hypertension.

3. Cirrhosis—Post-Sinusoidal Obstruction. When cirrhosis is severe it affects all parts of the liver anatomy and the fibrosis causes obstruction in the liver sinusoids and the draining hepatic veins. In these more serious cases of cirrhosis the liver function is abnormal. In addition the patient may have ascites.

C. Post-hepatic Observation

In this case the obstruction is in the hepatic veins or vena cava.

There is a rare disease in which the hepatic veins thrombose. This is called the Budd Chiari syndrome. Thrombosis of all the hepatic veins is not compatible with life but if one vein escapes the patient will survive with very severe effects of post-sinusoidal obstruction caused by obstruction to the venous outflow from most of the liver.

Post-hepatic obstruction always causes gross ascites.

Effects of Portal Hypertension

Collateral Formation

When there is an obstruction to the portal blood flow and a rise in portal pressure the body develops and enlarges branches of the portal vein to enable blood to flow away from the liver and to reach the vena cava by a route other than the normal one through the liver. These new veins are called collaterals and they are nature's way of trying to lower the portal pressure.

Sites of Collateral Vessels

The collateral vessels develop in several parts of the abdomen. Not all of these develop in every case.

Posterior abdominal wall veins. Tributaries of the splenic vein develop to carry blood into veins in the posterior abdominal wall, and these in turn drain into the inferior vena cava.

The umbilical vein may recanalize or a new vein may form near to the obliterated umbilical vein of the foetus. This carries portal blood from the main left hepatic vein to the region of the umbilicus where the veins join veins draining blood towards the heart. Sometimes these veins are visible round the umbilicus and this is called a 'caput medusae'.

There are other and complicated anatomical connections between the portal blood stream and the systemic veins. The most important is based on the coronary vein which drains blood from the portal vein into veins in the stomach and oesophagus. From these veins the blood passes to veins in the chest and so to the superior vena cava. As the pressure rises these veins greatly enlarge and bulge into the stomach and oesophagus where they have the appearance of varicose veins, and in consequence are called gastric and oesophageal varices (Fig. 27.2). This anastomosis helps to lower the portal pressure in the same way as the other anastomoses, but has the great disadvantage that serious haemorrhage may take place if they rupture into the stomach or oesophagus.

Splenomegaly

In cases of portal hypertension the spleen is enlarged as a result of the rise in pressure in the splenic vein which causes congestion of the spleen. When portal hypertension is relieved by a surgical operation the spleen becomes smaller.

29
Clinical Aspects of Portal Hypertension

There are two different clinical types of portal hypertension. One is concerned with pre-hepatic obstruction of the portal vein, and in these cases the liver function is normal. The second type concerns intra- and post-hepatic obstruction in which there is abnormal liver function. It follows that in many cases the signs and symptoms of cirrhosis will be present and they may dominate the clinical picture.

Pre-hepatic Obstruction

Many of these cases result from infection of the portal vein from the umbilicus in infancy. Portal hypertension develops early in life and the patient presents in childhood. The first clinical presentation is usually haematemesis resulting from rupture of oesophageal or gastric varices. Such bleeding may stop spontaneously but recurrence is usual unless steps are taken to lower the portal pressure.

As there is no liver disease the liver function tests are normal but because of raised venous pressure in the splenic vein there is obvious enlargement of the spleen. These patients are usually good operative risks but may die from haemorrhage from varices.

Intra-hepatic and Post-hepatic Obstruction

These patients may also present with gastro–oesophageal bleeding caused by rupture of varices. Again the bleeding may be severe enough to cause the patient's death. Splenic enlargement is observed on examination.

So far the patient presents a similar picture to the patient with pre-hepatic obstruction, but in addition there are the signs of intra-hepatic disease which is the cause of the portal hypertension. Sometimes a patient who is known to be cirrhotic is later admitted with a haematemesis.

Bilharzia

These patients usually come from the Middle East, in particular Egypt and Sudan, or from the Far East. Bilharzia is a serious disease and patients often have a haemoglobin level as low as 4 or 5 g and malnutrition. In addition, liver function is often severely affected so that these are very poor risk patients even after blood transfusion to restore the haemoglobin level. In late cases the liver is shrunken to less than half the normal size.

Cirrhosis

There are many causes of cirrhosis. In the world-wide picture malnutrition remains the most comon cause. Post-necrotic cirrhosis follows viral hepatitis, and in some parts of the world a high alcohol intake is an important causative factor. Patients with cirrhosis often have a large, hard liver, but in the later stages the liver is reduced in size.

When patients begin to show signs of liver failure there are certain clinical stigmata:

1. The palms of the hands are bright red (liver palms).
2. Spider naevi appear on the body. These are characterized by a central blood vessel which supplies the vessels of the naevus giving an appearance which has been likened to a spider (Fig. 29.1). When the central blood vessel is compressed the whole naevus blanches.

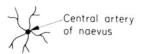

Fig. 29.1 Spider naevus.

3. There is often atrophy of the testes and enlargement of the breasts in the male.
4. In more severe cases there are signs in the central nervous system. There is a typical flapping tremor of the outstretched

hand, and eventually the patient goes into hepatic coma. These effects are often called portosystemic encephalopathy. In cirrhosis and portal hypertension there are natural shunts formed between the portal and the systemic circulations, and these enable products of digestion to bypass the liver and pass directly to the systemic circulation. They then pass to the brain causing the well-known symptoms. At one time ammonia was thought to be the main causative agent but this is no longer certain. Protein in the intestine exacerbates the symptoms, and serious encephalopathy and coma often follow a haemorrhage because of absorption of protein from the blood in the intestine. Sometimes encephalopathy appears after an operation to create a shunt. A shunt should be avoided if signs of encephalopathy are already present.

5. Ascites. Ascites is not a feature of portal hypertension and is never present in cases of pre-hepatic obstruction. The exact cause of ascites is unknown but it is related to cirrhosis with poor liver function, and is always present when the blood albumin is low. It is also a marked feature of post-sinusoidal obstruction and hepatic vein thrombosis.

Investigation of a Case of Portal Hypertension

Liver Function Tests

In cases of portal hypertension caused by cirrhosis it is important to assess liver function as this will affect the risk of certain types of operation for portal hypertension. The liver has great reserves of function and can regenerate after severe damage, so that the function tests may be normal in the presence of apparently severe cirrhosis. Many tests can be done, but those commonly done are described.

Blood Proteins

Albumin is made only in the liver. When liver function is impaired the albumin level in the blood falls. At the same time there may be an increase in the level of globulin in the blood. In a normal patient the albumin level is usually about double the globulin. In patients with cirrhosis the level of albumin and globulin may be equal or the ratio may be reversed with a higher level of globulin than albumin. Certain tests such as the thymol turbidity are positive when there is an excess of globulin, but the evaluation of different types of protein in the blood is now normally done with a test called paper chromatography.

Enzyme Studies

Serum glutamic oxaloacetic transaminase (SGOT) is normally present in a number of viscera including the heart and the liver. Damage to the cells of the heart or liver cause a rise in the level of SGOT, but the exact source is usually evident from the clinical history. A similar test is the serum glutamic pyruvic transaminase (SGPT) which is more specific for liver disease. In cases of hepatitis the tests show a considerable elevation because of the cell damage, but there is also some elevation in cases of cirrhosis.

Alkaline phosphatase is an enzyme which is concerned with normal function of bone and the blood level is always elevated in bone disease. Alkaline phosphatase is excreted by the liver into the bile, and any obstruction in the bile ducts within the liver or outside it causes an elevation of the alkaline phosphatase. Metastatic carcinoma is also associated with an elevated alkaline phosphatase.

Blood Bilirubin

Bilirubin is excreted in the bile by the liver. In patients with cirrhosis the bilirubin may be elevated.

Liver Biopsy

Liver biopsy is done by introducing a special needle into the liver with the object of removing a cylindrical-shaped fragment of tissue. The test is done under local anaesthetic. It is important to ask the patient to stop breathing during the procedure as the needle may tear the liver when the patient breathes.

The risk of this investigation is haemorrhage. It is usual to evaluate the patient's coagulation state before doing a liver biopsy and the test should not be done until the coagulation of the blood is normal. After the investigation it is important to make regular observations of the pulse rate and blood pressure. A rising pulse and falling blood pressure, especially if associated with sweating, suggests bleeding from the needle puncture of the liver, and the doctor should be called.

Scintillation Scanning

This test is absolutely without risk. Technetium sulphur colloid is injected. This substance is picked up by the reticulo-endothelial system, most of which is located in the liver. When the liver is scanned it is possible to identify non-functioning areas of over 2 cm in diameter.

Radiology

Barium studies are particularly useful in visualizing oesophageal varices.

Portal Venography

In this technique radio-opaque dye is introduced into the portal blood stream so that radiographs can be taken to demonstrate the anatomy of the portal venous system. Two techniques are in use:

1. The most common technique is to introduce a needle into the spleen under local anaesthetic (**Splenic portography**, see Fig. 29.2). A needle is introduced through the skin and placed

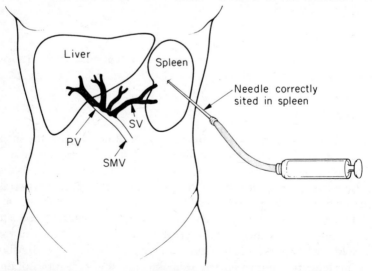

Fig. 29.2 Technique for splenic portography. The needle is placed within the spleen and X-rays taken immediately after injection of dye. PV, portal vein; SMV, superior mesenteric vein; SV, splenic vein.

in the centre of the spleen. The spleen is a very vascular organ and when the needle is properly located blood drips from the end. A syringe is then attached to the needle and the injection given. The films show the splenic and portal veins together with their tributaries and varices.

2. The second technique is **Transumbilical venography**. This can be used if the spleen has been removed or if the splenic vein is thrombosed. A small incision is made under local anaesthetic just above the umbilicus. The incision is explored until the surgeon finds the cord representing the obliterated umbilical vein. This can usually be incised and the obliterated lumen identified and re-opened with a probe. It joins the left branch of the portal vein, and once a backflow of blood is obtained a catheter can be passed into the portal vein and used for an injection of radio-opaque dye.

Oesophagoscopy

The new fibrelight instruments are much safer to use than the old metal and rigid oesophagoscopes. With these instruments it is easy to see varices in the oesophagus and stomach and also to see any associated gastric or duodenal ulcer.

30
Management of Bleeding from Gastro-oesophageal Varices

In most cases the differential diagnosis is between bleeding from a peptic ulcer or from varices. In children severe haematemesis is nearly always caused by rupture of varices. The history is helpful, and on examination enlargement of the spleen is particularly important. The signs of cirrhosis may also be present. If there is doubt about the diagnosis, and facilities exist, an oesophagoscopy and gastro-duodenoscopy should be done with the fibrescope. Some patients with varices turn out to be bleeding from an acute duodenal ulcer.

Blood Transfusion

As with any case of external or internal bleeding it is essential to replace blood lost and to transfuse sufficient blood to maintain a systolic blood pressure of 100 mm of mercury.

Pitressin

Pitressin is given intravenously. It acts by constricting the superior mesenteric artery and its branches and so reduces the flow of blood. This in turn reduces the flow in the mesenteric vein and lowers the portal blood pressure. A new development of this technique is to introduce a catheter into the mesenteric artery by the Seldinger technique. The pitressin can then be injected directly into the mesenteric artery where it is more effective as it has not been diluted.

Balloon Tamponade

If bleeding is not controlled by transfusion and pitressin some surgeons resort to tamponade using the Sengstaken tube. This tube has three channels (Fig. 30.1) and is passed into the stomach. One channel opens into the stomach and allows gastric drainage as with an ordinary gastric tube. The second channel inflates a balloon which should be located in the stomach. As the tube is withdrawn the stomach balloon cannot be pulled out of the stomach and is held up just below the oesophagus. With the stomach balloon in this position the third balloon is inflated. This balloon is placed just above the gastric balloon so that when it is inflated it will exert pressure on the oesophageal varices and control bleeding.

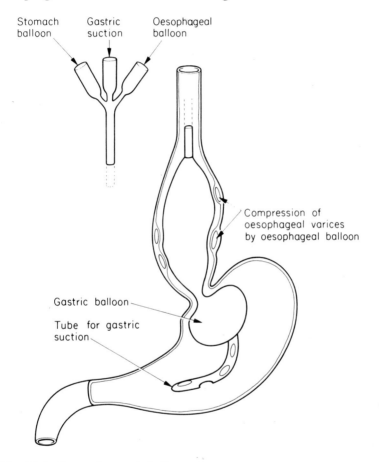

Fig. 30.1 Sengstaken triple balloon tube.

Nursing Care

The nursing care of the patient with an inflated balloon in the oesophagus is very difficult and important. No fluid may be given by mouth and the secretions from the salivary glands cannot be swallowed because the oesophagus is completely occluded by the balloon. There is a tendency for fluid to be regurgitated from the oesophagus and it may go into the trachea causing bronchitis and later pneumonitis. The patient is encouraged to spit out any secretions, and frequent suction is used on the mouth and pharynx.

The balloon is left in position for 48 hours. Unfortunately there is a considerable tendency for bleeding to recur when it is removed.

Emergency Surgery

If the patient continues to bleed in spite of conservative measures surgical treatment is considered.

Operations on the Varices

There are various operations which are directed to the varices which are ligated in the stomach or oesophagus. These operations are comparatively safe but do not lower the portal pressure. Recurrent bleeding is not uncommon.

Emergency Shunt Operations

An emergency shunt operation to lower the portal pressure and so stop bleeding from varices is a more serious undertaking. One reason for this is that the intestines are full of altered blood which is digested and absorbed into the portal blood stream. When the portal blood is shunted into the inferior vena cava this blood, containing the products of protein digestion, passes directly to the brain and may cause hepatic coma.

It is essential to use aperients and enemata to clear the blood from the bowel after an emergency shunt operation.

To overcome this dilemma some surgeons operate on the varices in an emergency to arrest bleeding and do an elective shunt three or four weeks later when the patient is not bleeding and is in better general condition.

31
Elective Treatment of Portal Hypertension

It must be emphasized that a history of bleeding from gastric or oesophageal varices is the only indication for surgical treatment of portal hypertension. Two distinct types of operative treatment may be undertaken.

1. Shunt Operations. There are a number of different operations, each of which is indicated in particular circumstances, in which the portal blood is diverted into a low-pressure systemic vein. In this way the portal pressure is reduced and varices become less tense so that rupture and haemorrhage are unlikely.

2. Operations on the Varices

1. Injection. Some surgeons inject oesophageal varices using an oesophagoscope. This is comparable with the injection treatment of varicose veins but is technically very much more difficult.
2. Operations on the stomach or oesophagus to ligate varices or to disconnect them from the high-pressure portal system. These operations are less risky than shunt operations and are indicated when liver function is poor. They are also indicated when suitable veins are not available for a shunt. The main disadvantage of operations on the varices is that while the portal hypertension persists there is a high risk of recurrence of the varices and further haemorrhage.

Porta–systemic Shunt Operations

The object of a shunt operation is to join a large vein in the portal circulation to a large vein in the systemic circulation. The effect of this is to lower the portal pressure by allowing free drainage into a low-pressure vein.

Indications

A history of severe oesophagogastric bleeding from varices is the only indication for a shunt. It is never done prophylactically simply because varices have been shown on an X-ray.

Liver function should be reasonably good and patients who have poor liver function are more safely treated by an operation on the varices.

It is essential to have good splenic portography to show the size and position of the main veins and to evaluate the possibility of doing a shunt.

Portacaval Shunt (Fig. 31.1)

This operation comprises a shunt between the portal vein and the inferior vena cava. Access is obtained through a right thoraco-abdominal incision or a long right subcostal incision. It is probably the most common shunt performed for portal hypertension.

The portal vein is identified and ligated where it divides into its right and left branches. The lower end of the portal vein is joined to the side of the inferior vena cava. In a few cases it is necessary to drain the hepatic end of the portal vein too and these cases are treated by double shunt or side to side anastomosis (Fig. 31.1).

Spleno-renal Shunt (Fig. 31.2)

The indications for this shunt are the same as for the portacaval shunt. It is particularly indicated when the portal vein is thrombosed or otherwise unsuitable for a shunt but the splenic vein remains patent. It is a more difficult operation than the portacaval shunt, and because of the smaller size of the veins which are anastomosed there is a greater tendency for the anastomosis to thrombose. However, because the shunt is smaller less intestinal blood is shunted to the systemic circulation and there is a lower risk of portasystemic encephalopathy.

The access is gained through a long left thoraco-abdominal inci-sion. The spleen is mobilized and removed and the splenic vein dissected free. The surgeon now turns to the renal vein which is situated at the back of the abdomen and a little lower down. It is usually possible to pick up a part of the renal vein in a special angled Satinsky clamp and to join the end of the splenic vein to the side of the renal vein. Complete clamping of the renal vein is undesirable as

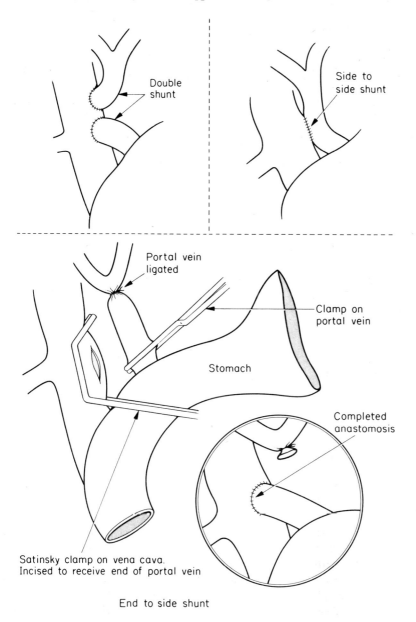

Double shunt

Side to side shunt

Portal vein ligated

Clamp on portal vein

Stomach

Completed anastomosis

Satinsky clamp on vena cava.
Incised to receive end of portal vein

End to side shunt

Fig. 31.1 End to side portacaval shunt.

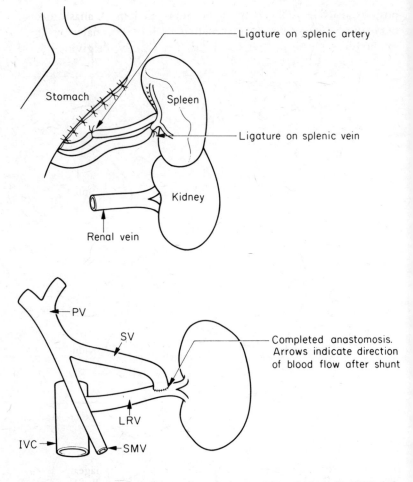

Fig. 31.2 Splenorenal shunt. PV, portal vein; SV, splenic vein; LRV, left renal vein; IVC, inferior vena cava; SMV, superior mesenteric vein.

the kidney will be permanently damaged if its circulation is arrested for more than 20 minutes.

Distal Spleno-renal Anastomosis (Warren)

This operation is theoretically the best shunt but is unfortunately technically very difficult. Some surgeons always do this operation when a shunt is indicated. The object of the operation is to drain the gastric and oesophageal varices through the spleen which is left in position and then to the systemic system by making an anastomosis of the splenic end of the splenic vein to the side of the renal vein. This can best be understood by reference to Fig. 31.3. While giving good

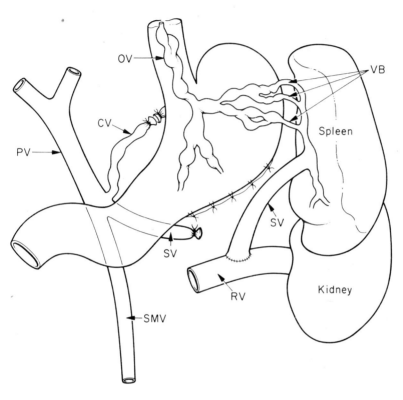

Fig. 31.3 Distal splenorenal shunt (Warren). OV, oesophageal varices; VB, basa brevia; PV, portal vein; CV, coronary vein (ligated); SV, splenic vein; SMV, superior mesenteric vein; RV, renal vein.

decompression of the varices the operation does not involve shunting of intestinal blood into the systemic system so that theoretically there is no risk of porta-systemic encephalopathy.

Superior Mesenteric—Inferior Vena Cava Shunt (Mesocaval Shunt)

When the patient's life is threatened by repeated haemorrhage from varices but the previously described shunts are technically impossible, the surgeon may be able to do a shunt between the superior

mesenteric vein and the inferior vena cava. This operation is particularly indicated when the portal and splenic veins are thrombosed, or
when the portal vein is thrombosed and the splenic vein lost through
an ill advised splenectomy.

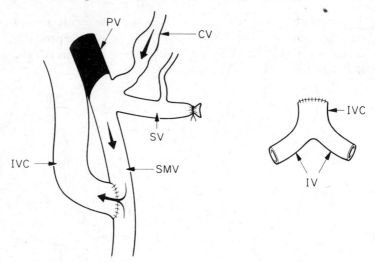

Fig. 31.4 Mesocaval shunt. CV, coronary vein; PV, portal vein (thrombosed); SV, splenic vein; IVC, inferior vena cava; SMV, superior mesenteric
vein; IV, iliac vein.

This operation may stop bleeding from varices and so save the
patient's life, but it has two serious drawbacks. The intestinal blood
is shunted directly into the vena cava, so giving a high risk of
porta-systemic encephalopathy. The second difficulty concerns the
fact that to accomplish the anastomosis it is necessary to ligate the
inferior vena cava. This often causes considerable swelling of the legs
and quite a lot of disability. The operation is best understood by
reference to Fig. 31.4. An alternative and easier technique is to use a
short, wide (20 mm) Dacron graft (H graft) to connect the inferior
vena cava to the mesenteric vein.

Post-operative Observations

The general observations needed in any major abdominal operation
are applied. In addition it is important to watch for changes in the
state of consciousness or confusion which may indicate the onset of
encephalopathy.

Operations on the Varices

Porta-systematic Disconnection

This operation was first described by Tanner and is sometimes referred to by his name. The operation is probably the procedure of choice in patients suffering from schistosomiasis. In this condition a splenectomy is often performed at the same time.

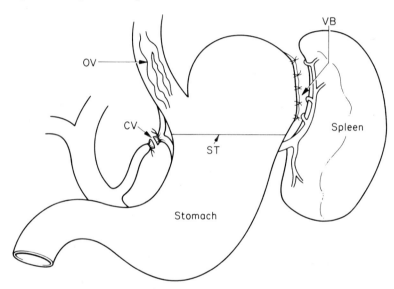

Fig. 31.5 Portasystemic disconnection (Tanner). OV, oesophageal varices; CV, coronary vein divided; ST, stomach transection; VB, vasa brevia divided.

There are three steps in the operation which are shown in Fig. 31.5. The operation is usually performed through an upper abdominal incision.

1. To ligate and divide the coronary vein.
2. To divide the vasa brevia. These are the vessels running between the upper part of the stomach and the spleen.
3. To transect the stomach and to resuture it.

These three steps effectively disconnect the varices in the oesophagus and upper part of the stomach from the portal system. In spite of this many patients get recurrent varices which bleed again.

Ligation of Oesophageal Varices

Access to the oesophagus requires a thoracotomy and this is usually done by resecting part of the eighth rib. The oesophagus is identified and mobilized from its bed. Two light clamps are put on the oesophagus to prevent bleeding from varices when it is incised, then a longitudinal incision about 7 cm long is made into the oesophagus. The longitudinally running varices are then seen inside the oesophagus and each of these is oversewn with a continuous catcut suture. The oesophagus is closed with interrupted non–absorbable material and the chest closed with a thoracotomy drain connected to an underwater seal.

The recently introduced stapling gun has been used to simplify this operation. After division of the veins leading to the oesophagus the intra-abdominal part of the oesophagus is immobilized. The stapling gun is introduced into the oesophagus through an incision in the stomach. When the gun is fired by pulling the trigger a circular blade cuts through the oesophagus and the ends are immediately secured together with an encircling row of metal staples. In this way the oesophagus and its varices are divided and accurately sutured without the need to open the chest.

Post-operative observation and management

The shunt operations on the varices are subject to similar problems and can be considered together.

1. Thoracotomy. If the chest has been opened a chest X-ray is taken in the recovery room. This is to ensure that the lung is fully inflated.

There will be a chest drain and this is connected to an underwater seal. So long as the tube is not blocked there will be oscillation of the level of water in the tube with respiration. Any discharge of blood should be measured as it collects in the bottle. Discharge of bubbles of air should be noted and reported.

2. Laparotomy. When there has been a major operation in the abdomen there is a tendency for the intestines to stop working for a time. The patient will need gastric suction with a Ryles tube and the aspirate must be collected, measured, and charted. Because there is no oral intake the patient will receive intravenous fluid until the intestinal function returns.

3. Urine output. Measurement of urine output is very important as it is an indication of the state of hydration and of renal function. It is usual to manage patients with an in-dwelling catheter so that the output can be accurately measured.

4. Hepatic coma. There is an increased risk of hepatic coma particularly following shunt operations. Observations on the patient's general state of consciousness and possible mental confusion should be reported to the doctor.

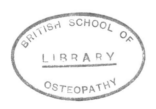

Glossary

Acute   Something of sudden onset.

Anaesthetic   When this word is used in reference to a part of the body it means that there is no sensation in that part.

Anaphylaxis   A severe and dangerous reaction of the body to the introduction of a drug or poison.

Ankle jerk   When the tendon at the back of the ankle (Achilles tendon) is tapped the calf muscle reacts by contracting. The ankle jerk is absent if the nerve pathways are not working.

Anticoagulants   Drugs which prevent coagulation of the blood.

Arteriogram   An X-ray of the arteries which are shown after an injection of radio-opaque fluid directly into the artery.

Atherosclerosis   A generalized disease of the arteries in which plaques of yellow fatty material are deposited in the wall resulting in narrowing and irregularity.

Atrial septal defect   An abnormal opening in the septum which separates the right and left atria of the heart.

Caput medusae   In Greek mythology Medusa had a head of snakes. The term is used to refer to large veins radiating from the umbilicus and is seen in some cases of portal hypertension.

Catalyst   A substance which increases the speed of a reaction

Chiropodist   A person who gives treatment to affections of the foot.

Chronic   Long continued illness.

Claudication, intermittent   Pain in the leg on walking. It is typical that the pain is relieved by stopping walking.

Collateral   Alternative blood vessels which develop as a natural attempt to overcome an arterial occlusion.

Dacron   A man-made fire used for making sutures and artificial arteries for grafting.

Dextran   A solution made by joining molecules of dextrose. Used in emergency treatment of shock.

Distal   Furthest away.

Embolectomy   An operation at which an embolus is removed.

Embolus   A body, usually a blood clot, which travels in the blood stream and causes obstruction to the circulation at the point its progress is arrested.

Endarterectomy   An operation in which an atherosclerotic occlusion is removed.

Endothelium   The inner lining of a blood vessel.

Fibrillation (Atrial)   A condition of the atria of the heart in which they do not contract properly and effectively.

Ganglion   A collection of nerve cells causing a swelling on a nerve.

Gangrene   Death of tissue with infection and putrefaction.

Hemiplegia   Paralysis of one side of the body.

Heparin   A drug which prevents coagulation of the blood.

Hyperaemia   An increase in the blood supply to a part of the body.

Image intensifier   An electronic device for brightening the X-ray screen image. The image is displayed on a television screen.

Ischaemia   Reduction in the blood supply.

Ketone   A substance which is present in the blood and urine in patients with diabetes mellitus.

Laminated   In layers like the substance of an onion.

Metabolism   The living processes of cells.

Mitral valve   Valve in the heart between the left atrium and the left ventricle preventing reflux of blood.

Haematoma   A collection of blood in the tissues, forming a lump.

Hamartoma   A lump consisting of a local malformation of tissue.

Necrosis   Death of tissue.

Paraesthesia   Abnormal sensations.

Platelets   Small cells circulating in the blood stream and connected with coagulation of the blood.

Proximal   Nearest.

Sympathectomy   Removal of sympathetic nerves.

Sympathetic nerve   Nerves controlling function of the viscera and blood vessels.

Tamponade   Compression from outside. Often refers to compression of the heart.

Teflon   A man-made substance used to cover metal to make it inert in the body.

Telangiectasis   An area of dilated capillaries appearing as a small red spot.

Toxic   Poisonous to the body.

Trauma   Injury.

Tricuspid valve   Valve between the right atrium and right ventricle preventing reflux of blood.

Vibration sense   The ability of the patient to feel a vibrating tuning fork placed in contact with the body.

Index